NEARLY 40 MILLION AMERICANS HAVE HIGH BLOOD PRESSURE. IT CAN THREATEN ANYONE, AT ANY AGE. UNTREATED, IT CAN LEAD TO STROKE, HEART ATTACK AND OTHER SERIOUS ILLNESSES. IN ALMOST EVERY CASE, HIGH BLOOD PRESSURE *CAN* BE SUCCESSFULLY TREATED.

The Pill Book of High Blood Pressure, written especially for the consumer, tells you everything you should know about the medications doctors prescribe for the treatment of hypertension. Here is the information right at your fingertips, including cautions and warnings, side effects, adverse reactions, usual dosage levels, and the potential for overdose. PLUS the causes and dangers of high blood pressure, and how to live successfully with hypertension.

D0711412

The purpose of this book is to provide educational information to the public concerning the drugs most commonly prescribed by physicians for the treatment of high blood pressure. It is not intended to be complete or exhaustive or in any respect a substitute for personal medical care. *Only a physician may prescribe these drugs and the exact dosage that should be taken.*

While every effort has been made to reproduce products on the cover and insert of this book in an exact fashion, certain variations of size or color may be expected as a result of the photographic process. Furthermore, pictures identified as brand-name drugs should not be confused with their generic counterparts, and vice versa. *In any event, the reader should not rely on the photographic image to identify any pills depicted herein, but should rely solely on the physician's prescription as dispensed by the pharmacist.*

THE PILL BOOK OF HIGH BLOOD PRESSURE

BERT STERN

Producer

LAWRENCE D. CHILNICK

Editor-in-Chief

TEXT BY

R. C. Garrett

U. G. Waldmeyer

MEDICAL CONSULTANT
Harold S. Solomon, M.D.
Assistant Professor of Medicine,
Harvard Medical School

ADDITIONAL TEXT / PRODUCTION
Daniel Montopoli

BANTAM BOOKS
TORONTO • NEW YORK • LONDON • SYDNEY • AUCKLAND

*Special acknowledgment to Tom Holdorf
for photography assistance.*

*Special thanks to Jeff Packer
and Dave Phillips, Carlyle Chemists,
New York City.*

THE PILL BOOK OF HIGH BLOOD PRESSURE
A Bantam Book / March 1985

ISBN 0-553-24489-2

Published simultaneously in the United States and Canada

*Bantam Books are published by Bantam Books, Inc. Its
trademark, consisting of the words ''Bantam Books'' and the
portrayal of a rooster, is Registered in U.S. Patent and Trademark Office and in other countries. Marca Registrada. Bantam Books, Inc., 666 Fifth Avenue, New York, New York
10103.*

PRINTED IN THE UNITED STATES OF AMERICA

O   0 9 8 7 6 5 4 3 2 1

Contents

HOW TO USE THIS BOOK

The Pill Book of High Blood Pressure is divided into three main sections:

I. Information about the many aspects of high blood pressure, including details about the nature of the disease, treatments both medical and non-traditional, and facts you should know about living with high blood pressure.

II. Easy-to-read profiles of the drugs most often prescribed to treat high blood pressure.

III. Life-sized pictures of the hypertension drugs most commonly prescribed in the United States.

The Pill Book of High Blood Pressure's photo system for checking medications is designed to help you quickly identify the drug you're about to take. Included are the most popular brand-name drugs, and many of the drugs most frequently prescribed by generic name. Although several dosage levels may be included, other dosage levels may be omitted because they are prescribed less often.

The drugs are organized alphabetically and have been reproduced as faithfully as possible. While every effort has been made to depict the drugs accurately, certain variations in size and color must be expected as a result of the photographic and printing processes. Therefore, you should never rely solely on the photographic image to identify any pill, but should check with your doctor or pharmacist if you have any questions whatsoever about the identification.

Most, but not all, of the drugs in the color section can be matched with your high blood pressure medication by matching your pill with the following on each photo:

• The imprinted company logo (e.g., "Lilly," "Roche")
• The product strength (e.g., "250 mg.," "10 mg.")
• The product code number, which may be imprinted on the pill

Because many generic drugs look the same as their brand-name counterparts, some manufacturers have started printing the product name on each pill.

To find out more about the drug shown, check the descriptive text on the pages referred to in the photo caption. The pill profiles provide complete descriptions of the most often prescribed generic and brand-name high blood pressure drugs. The descriptions give you detailed information about your prescriptions. The easy-to-read profiles are listed alphabetically by their generic names (except when the product profiled is a combination of two or more generic drugs; in which case, the popular brand names for these combinations are profiled in alphabetical order).

The drug profiles contain the following information:

Generic Name: The generic name is the drug's common name, or chemical name, as approved by the Food and Drug Administration (FDA).

Brand Name(s): The brand name is the name

given by a particular drug company to identify its product. For example, Inderal is a brand name for the generic drug propranolol hydrochloride. When particular drugs are also sold under their generic names, that information is included here.

Ingredients: The ingredients are listed whenever a high blood pressure medication is a combination of two or more generic drugs.

Type of Drug: How the individual drug is classified, which may indicate its relation to other drugs. For example, Lopressor, classed as a beta blocker, is closely related to other beta blockers such as Corgard, Visken, and Inderal. More information about these drug types is provided at the beginning of section II.

Prescribed for: The condition for which a drug is most often prescribed.

Cautions and Warnings: Any drug can be harmful if you are sensitive to any of its actions. The information provided here alerts you to possible allergic reactions, and to certain personal physical conditions, such as pregnancy and diabetes, which should be taken into consideration if the drug is prescribed for you.

Possible Side Effects: These are the more common side effects to be expected from the drug.

Possible Adverse Effects: Less common effects of a pill that may be cause for concern. If you are not sure whether you are experiencing an adverse reaction, ALWAYS CALL YOUR DOCTOR.

Drug Interactions: This section tells you what other drugs should be avoided when taking the hypertension pills. Drug interactions with other pills, alcohol, food, or other substances can cause death. Interactions are more common than overdoses. It is very important to be careful when drinking alcohol with any medication, or when taking several drugs at the same time. Be sure to inform your doctor of any medication—prescription or nonprescription—you have been taking. Your pharmacist should also keep a record of all your prescriptions and over-the-counter drugs. This listing, generally called a Patient Drug Profile, is used to review your record should problems arise. You may want to keep your own record and bring it to your pharmacist for review whenever a new medicine is added.

Usual Dose: The maximum and minimum amounts of a drug that are usually prescribed. However, you may be given different dosage instructions by your doctor. It is important to check with your doctor if you are confused about how often to take a pill, and when, or if you have been given a dosage different from that indicated in this book. You should not change the prescribed dosage of any drug you are taking without first talking to your doctor.

Overdosage: The symptoms of a drug overdose and the immediate steps you should take if overdose occurs are detailed whenever there is a danger of an overdose reaction.

If you read something in *The Pill Book of High Blood Pressure* that does not coincide with your doctor's instructions, call your doctor, who may have had special reasons for prescribing different medications, or different dosages from those referred to here.

Any drug can have serious side effects if used improperly or abused. We advise you to learn all you can about the drugs you're taking—the benefits and dangers alike.

I
High Blood Pressure in the 1980s

1.

WHAT IS HIGH BLOOD PRESSURE?

High blood pressure:
- *Has no symptoms*
- *Can threaten anyone, at any age*
- *Is a very serious illness*
- *Can cause strokes and heart attacks*
- *Can be treated effectively*

Nearly 40,000,000 Americans—*40 million!*—have high blood pressure.

That's roughly one out of every six men, women, and children across the country. For those who already know they have high blood pressure, which doctors call "hypertension," there's good news today. In almost every case, it can be successfully treated by the wise use of a variety of medications and other relatively simple procedures.

But there is ample reason for high blood pressure to be known as "the silent killer." Many of its victims are unaware that they have hypertension, and if left untreated, it can lead to strokes, heart attacks, and other serious ailments.

In America, physicians diagnose and treat hypertension more than any other chronic disease. It is being uncovered in the course of routine insurance checkups, during elaborate physicals of famous television actors and actresses, by military doctors performing standard tests on seemingly healthy recruits, and even during checkups of toddlers by their pediatricians (yes, youngsters can have hypertension, too).

High blood pressure is not restricted to the United States. Around the world, a substantial percentage of the population has hypertension. It is a condition striking all races, ages, and religions. Economic and political barriers do not exist for high blood pressure either. Hypertension is more prevalent in some nations than in others, but globally as many as *900 million* individuals may have high blood pressure.

So common—and so dangerous—is high blood pressure that it is viewed by specialists as a major factor in the deaths of at least 250,000 Americans annually. Around the world, high blood pressure may play a role in the premature deaths of more than 100 million people every year.

It's as though each month, the entire population of a major city like New York, Paris, Peking, or Moscow disappears from the face of the earth. The loss is not only staggering but needless.

In recent years, hypertension—once a mystery to doctors and laymen alike—has become easy to diagnose and simple to treat. Dozens of drugs have been developed that lower blood pressure and dramatically reduce the risk of disability and premature death. When used according to a physician's instructions, these medications can save millions of lives.

These medications include drugs that lower blood pressure by reducing the amount of liquid in the body, drugs that open the blood vessels wider and let blood circulate freely under less pressure, and drugs that lower the force with which the heart pumps blood. These medications have already saved the lives of millions of people, and can save millions more if their hypertension is discovered before it causes permanent damage to their bodies.

What Is Blood Pressure?

---

* Measuring blood pressure is easy and painless
* Blood pressure must be checked regularly
* There are accepted norms for blood pressure
* It is normal for blood pressure to vary through the day, and from one day to another

---

If you prick your finger, a droplet of blood will probably appear within a few seconds. The blood pushes out of the injury because it is under pressure, much like water in a garden hose. If the hose has a leak, the pressurized water will squirt out. Similarly, the pressure of blood will force it out through a wound.

Inside your body, the pressure is generated by your heart. It rhythmically squeezes blood into your arteries throughout your life. The pressure generated by your heart is, of course, much lower than that provided by a garden hose. But it is sufficient in a healthy person to push blood through nearly 100,000 miles of blood vessels, from large ones about the size of your finger, down to vessels so minuscule that blood cells must squeeze through one at a time.

With every heartbeat, a surge of pressure pulses into your blood vessels. Physicians call this pressure surge "systolic," from the Greek word for "contraction," which is precisely what your heart does each time it beats.

There is a second kind of blood pressure within your body, which occurs in the moments between heartbeats. It is caused by the elasticity of your blood vessels as they push back against the blood your heart just forced into them. This pressure is called "diastolic," from the Greek word meaning "expansion."

Systolic pressure, then, is the force with which your heart pumps blood; diastolic pressure is the force of your blood vessels on the blood.

How Blood Pressure Is Measured

Doctors measure the systolic and diastolic pressure with a device that records how high the pressure of your heart and arteries would lift a glass-enclosed column of mercury. However, actual glass tubes of mercury are almost never used today, having been replaced by highly accurate pressure gauges.

While most people rely on physicians or experienced medical technicians to measure their blood pressure, increasing numbers of men and women are checking themselves for hypertension. The equipment most often used—a sphygmomanometer, or sphyg (pronounced "sfig") for short—consists of a hollow, inflatable cuff, a pressure gauge, and a stethoscope. It is available to anyone through medical-supply stores or by mail from various firms, most of which provide complete instructions for its use.

The cuff is wrapped around the upper arm and inflated until, like a tourniquet, it stops the flow of blood through the brachial artery, which lies just under the skin above the inside of the elbow.

Pressure is then slowly reduced until blood circulation resumes. When blood again begins to flow through the artery, loud thumping noises can be heard through the stethoscope. The pressure indicated on the gauge when the sound of circulation resumes is the systolic pressure.

As the cuff continues to deflate, the sound grows fainter because the blood is flowing more easily. At the exact moment the sound stops, the pressure indicated on the gauge is the diastolic pressure.

The two readings are usually noted together, as though they're a fraction. So, a blood pressure reading of "120 millimeters of mercury systolic, over 80 millimeters of mercury diastolic," is usually written simply "120/80" and referred to as "120 over 80."

What the Numbers Mean

After years of studying blood-pressure statistics around the world and conducting extensive research throughout the United States, researchers have determined blood pressure "averages" that are almost universally accepted.

At any reading above "normal," you run an increased risk of dying prematurely of heart disease, stroke, or one of a number of other ailments, if the higher pressure is continuous. High blood pressure, though, even at the "severely hypertensive" level, does not itself cause death. That's right—hypertension does not kill. Instead, it *causes* the conditions that *do* kill.

Although researchers have yet to pinpoint the exact way in which hypertension leads to so many ailments, statistical evidence clearly shows that life expectancy is shortened—sometimes dramatically—by high blood pressure.

An average person diagnosed at age 35 as having mild to moderate hypertension can expect to live only to about 60, if the high blood pressure is not treated. The same individual with normal blood pressure can expect to live to 76. Thus, untreated hypertension can cut as much as sixteen years from life.

Even with borderline hypertension—a diastolic reading of about 92 or 93—your life span can be shortened. Statistically, untreated hypertension in this range can reduce life expectancy by two to four years.

Of course, some people with mild or moderate hypertension will always live longer than statistics indicate. But those who beat the odds are truly rare. Would you want to take the chance of losing more than a decade of your own life?

BLOOD PRESSURE READINGS

If your systolic pressure is:	And your diastolic pressure is:	You are:
100–140	70–90	normal (the majority of people)
140–159	90–94	mildly hypertensive
160–179	94–114	moderately hypertensive
180–up	115–up	severely hypertensive

Healthy Blood Pressure

Many things can alter your blood pressure; it seldom remains the same from one minute to the next.

As you change your level of activity—by standing up, walking around, or sitting down—your heart beats harder and faster or slower and less powerfully. When you sleep, your blood pressure drops considerably, and if you sleep through the night, it probably reaches its lowest level at about 3:00 or 4:00 A.M.

When you are startled—a loud noise might be sufficient—your blood pressure rises suddenly, then usually falls again when you realize there is no real danger. It also changes according to your level of stress or anxiety. If you are worried about meeting a deadline at work, your blood pressure will probably go up temporarily. Similarly, the death of a close friend or family member can raise your blood pressure.

Such pressure fluctuations are due partly to changes in the level of various hormones and other chemicals in your body, which tell your heart to "speed up a little," or "slow down, danger has passed."

Body chemical and electrical impulses also deliver instructions to your blood vessels; for instance: "Tighten up your arm and leg vessels, so more blood can go to your heart and brain."

These signals are transmitted by hormones like epinephrine and norepinephrine (also called adrenaline)—which are manufactured by the adrenal glands on top of your kidneys—and by pressure-sensitive cells in your body called "baroreceptors," which are part of your nervous system.

Baroreceptors act like electronic thermostats. They tell your body when to raise or lower blood pressure, depending on the needs of different parts of your body for a greater or lesser amount of blood. The most important group of baroreceptors is situated just where the carotid artery, which carries blood to your brain, forms a branch in your neck.

Another substance, called renin, is produced by your kidneys whenever blood pressure drops. The renin, in turn, creates a hormone called angiotensin, which tightens your arteries and thus raises your blood pressure. The angiotensin also stimulates the release of yet another hormone, aldosterone, which further regulates blood pressure.

The multiple body systems that control blood pressure are, for the most part, fully automatic. You don't have to concentrate on making your heart beat harder or faster when you're walking in the woods, say, and encounter a dangerous animal. Your body automatically gives you the balance of heartbeat and blood flow that makes your escape easiest.

When you meet a dangerous animal or even a threatening business associate—during any emergency, in fact—it is completely normal for your blood pressure to rise. Such increases are not part of the medical diagnosis of hypertension. Much more important is your basic blood pressure when you are resting, for instance while relaxing at home.

Emergencies raise blood pressure for only a few minutes at a time, and your body can easily cope with such temporary jumps. But your blood pressure when you're relaxing should not be so high that your system must constantly overwork just to circulate your blood.

Signs and Signals

As we have seen, any blood pressure reading above 140/90 is considered dangerous.

Unfortunately, high blood pressure almost never produces symptoms until it is so far advanced that major damage has already been done to the cardiovascular system, the kidneys, or some other part of the body. The only way to know whether you have hypertension is to have your blood pressure checked.

If any symptoms are present, the most common one is a headache, usually occurring in the morning and disappearing as the day wears on. A handful of hypertensive individuals encounter unexpected fatigue, irritation, and nervousness; and a few complain of dizziness, faintness, or a subtle pressure in the chest. But it is extremely difficult to recognize any of these signals by yourself, and they can be the result of any number of other ailments.

Since blood pressure fluctuates frequently throughout the day, doctors prefer taking several readings before making a diagnosis. There is always the possibility that a single high reading is the result of nervousness on visiting the physician or is due to a particularly rough day at work. Most doctors will ask you to return another day for additional blood-pressure tests prior to suggesting hypertension medications or other treatment.

2.

WHAT CAUSES HIGH BLOOD PRESSURE?

- *Your habits can contribute to high blood pressure*
- *So can your personality*
- *Even the environment may be partly responsible*
- *High blood pressure may be hereditary, too*

Secondary Hypertension

There are two types of high blood pressure, which physicians have termed "essential" and "secondary."

Secondary hypertension can be found in about 3 to 5 percent of those with high blood pressure. This type of hypertension has a distinct, known cause, and if the underlying cause is corrected, blood pressure usually returns to normal.

Any number of kidney ailments can cause hypertension by interfering with the normal production of the hormone renin. Other diseases—including damage to the artery that brings blood to the kidneys—can alter blood pressure throughout the body.

Small tumors can also cause high blood pressure, as can various chemical imbalances in the body.

Birth-control pills can bring about secondary hypertension. Usually, if the blood pressure is only slightly elevated, merely stopping the use of the pills brings pressure back to normal. In some cases, however, other factors contribute to the hypertension, and it fails to stop even after the pills are discontinued. At that point it is considered "essential" hypertension, and additional treatment is required.

In many cases, secondary hypertension can be cured by surgery, or by the use of drugs treating the ailment that caused the elevation of blood pressure.

Essential Hypertension

LINKS TO ESSENTIAL HYPERTENSION

- *Heredity*
- *Overweight*
- *Inactive lifestyle*
- *Dietary factors including salt and cholesterol*
- *Stress*

Essential hypertension is the most common type of high blood pressure, affecting an estimated 95 to 97 percent of those who have the illness.

No one knows precisely what causes essential hypertension. Unlike infection (which stems from an invasion of your body by something that can be seen and identified under a microscope), essential hypertension is an illness of regulation, during which one or more body mechanisms simply stop their normal clockwork task of maintaining proper blood pressure.

This does not mean, however, that doctors are ignorant about essential hypertension. They know with certainty, for example, that several factors, including many you can control, play a role in high blood pressure. And they know that by lowering blood pressure, people will live longer.

Physicians call the factors contributing to hypertension "risk factors" because each presents an increased risk that anyone falling into certain groups will develop the disease.

Heredity

Just as gray eyes or curly hair can run in families, so can high blood pressure.

Particular physical traits—a curved or straight nose, a tall or short body—seldom appear in every family member, but instead are seen in only one parent, perhaps, or maybe an uncle, a grandmother, or a sibling.

Similarly, high blood pressure seldom occurs in every member of a family. But studies show that if one parent has hypertension, there is a good chance that one out of every four children will develop the illness. And if both parents have high blood pressure, it is likely that half their children will, too.

While many of the physical characteristics passed on from parents to children are tied to a single gene, hypertension is probably influenced by several genes. When a certain combination of genetic information is in place, an individual will be predisposed to high blood pressure. Some experts estimate that heredity is the primary cause for fully one-third of all hypertension cases.

This does not mean that heredity automatically spells trouble. Some people with a family history of hypertension will never develop the disease, even if they fit into every risk category leading to high blood pressure. And many others will develop hypertension even when they seem not to be genetically predisposed.

However, if several members of your family have been diagnosed as hypertensive, or have been stricken by one or another of the illnesses often brought on by high blood pressure (heart disease or heart failure, atherosclerosis, stroke, kidney failure), you should make sure all family members, no matter how healthy they look and feel, are checked for hypertension.

The earlier a diagnosis is made and treatment begins, the less damage will be done to the body's vital blood-supply system.

Overweight

Overweight people face a considerable risk of developing high blood pressure. Furthermore, if you were overweight as a youngster, even if you have lost weight since then, you are still in danger of becoming hypertensive.

In adult life, almost any weight gain of more than a few pounds tends to increase blood pressure. If the pressure was already in the hypertensive range, even a slight increase can be threatening to your health.

Overweight and obesity (significant overweight) are common conditions in America. A large percentage of people gain weight as they grow older, and their blood pressures rise at the same time. This is true regardless of height, sex, or age.

Comparisons have been made between overweight people in the United States and in less-developed countries, and the corresponding cases of high blood pressure. The studies show clearly that excessive weight is closely linked to hypertension.

How excess weight affects the circulation of blood can be explained easily. Your heart must pump blood to the most remote parts of your body all day, every day of your life. The blood must nourish not only your kidneys, liver, brain, lungs, and muscles—to say nothing of skin and countless other organs—but also any fat cells you may have. For the heart to pump blood to just ten extra pounds of fat requires it to work substantially harder; imagine the strain on your heart if it is called upon to pump blood to an extra fifty pounds of fat! Not everyone who is overweight, of course, has high blood pressure, but the statistical link exists.

Weight reduction not only eases the heart's burden but reduces blood pressure at the same time. In one study of severely overweight people with hypertension, their blood pressures dropped significantly when they lost even a few pounds.

Another study linking overweight to hypertension was conducted on almost 550 men and women in their teens and twenties. Those who were overweight when they were young registered higher blood pressures fifteen years later, along with increased instances of other illnesses and a higher death rate.

But not everyone who is overweight has high blood pressure, and researchers are still trying to understand the precise ways in which extra weight causes hypertension. For the moment, though, it is enough to recognize that the cause-and-effect relationship exists.

Lack of Exercise

If you are physically inactive—for instance, if you work in a quiet office, don't get out much, and watch TV for hours every evening—your chances of developing high blood pressure increase.

Virtually every hypertension study comparing sedentary people with those who exercise regularly shows that exercise lowers blood pressure.

It is unclear whether the exercise alone is responsible for the lower rate of hypertension, or the weight loss that usually accompanies exercise is more important. But there is little question that the easy life is not necessarily the healthy life.

Some researchers believe that improved muscle tone helps the body move blood through arteries and veins, and that for this reason alone, exercise is a vital component in warding off hypertension.

Diet

SALT is the most-talked-about dietary substance that experts connect to hypertension. But is it really a risk factor? The scientific evidence is inconclusive.

Within the medical community there are strong opinions on both sides of a growing controversy: "Yes, using excessive salt leads to hypertension," and, "No, salt has nothing to do with high blood pressure."

Table salt is sodium chloride, 40 percent of which is sodium, an element required by the body. Sodium helps the body retain fluids, and a higher fluid level leads to greater blood volume. Usually, this would increase blood pressure.

But many studies show little or no difference in hypertension rates between those who use a minimum of salt and those who use significantly larger amounts. Other studies indicate no notable reduction in high blood pressure when patients eliminate or reduce their salt intake.

One comprehensive British study attempted to determine whether the children of hypertensive parents could lower their chances of having high blood pressure by altering salt intake when still young. But even that study ended without clear results, leaving it questionable whether salt causes high blood pressure or hypertension causes an increased desire for salt.

Nevertheless, while the debate continues, most physicians agree that for people who are genetically predisposed to high blood pressure, or for those who fall into any of the other risk categories, it is wise to eliminate as much salt as possible from the diet.

CHOLESTEROL has consistently been blamed for producing high blood pressure, or at least for making hypertension more likely, by scores of medical researchers.

Indeed, the fatty deposits that build up inside blood vessels and reduce the flow of blood through the body are composed primarily of cholesterol. And cholesterol is a basic component of much of the food we Americans love to eat, including eggs, butter, and beef.

CALCIUM insufficiency, similarly, has been linked to hypertension. Calcium plays an important role in regulating the rate and force of heartbeats and the way electrical signals reach the muscles. Some doctors urge their hypertensive patients to eat more calcium-rich foods as one step toward lowering blood pressure. The real link is still being established.

Stress

There is no doubt that stress, at work or at home, can cause significant increases in blood pressure.

Usually, however, such increases are temporary. When the cause of the stress is eliminated—the boss calms down, the kids clean up their room, the air-conditioner is finally fixed—blood pressure returns to normal. A healthy individual can easily withstand repeated temporary bouts of stress-related hypertension. It is prolonged stress that causes trouble.

The effects of long-term stress on blood pressure have been demonstrated in studies of men and women exposed consistently to high pressure in their work.

One well-researched group is the air-traffic controllers, who are responsible for the lives of millions of air travelers. At airports where air traffic is particularly heavy, controllers have a much higher than normal hypertension rate. Where air traffic is low, hypertension rates are also low.

Personality

Not everyone who experiences constant stress develops high blood pressure. The key to avoiding hypertension in a stressful environment may be your personality type. Experts have divided people into two personality categories, depending on the way they handle stress.

Those who feel a constant sense of competitiveness and always seem rushed for time—traits common among business leaders—are classified as Type A personalities. They often view everyday events as emergencies, and their bodies respond by increasing the heart rate and raising the blood pressure. Such Type A responses to stress can be found in any group, not just business executives. To develop hypertension, Type A's generally must also simultaneously face some other risk factors.

Type B personalities, on the other hand, seem to care little about "getting ahead" and appear unconcerned about being on time for appointments. Their blood pressures are usually lower, and, ironically, they may in the long run achieve more than their hard-driving Type A counterparts because of their increased life expectancy.

Environment

Environmental factors such as cigarette smoke have been statistically linked to hypertension. For someone who has high blood pressure and who smokes, the chances of stroke are *sixteen times* greater than for a hypertensive who does not smoke. Air pollution and excessive noise, however, have not been decisively tied to high blood pressure.

Race

Hypertension is the leading reason why blacks have a shorter life expectancy than whites.

A black American has a 50 percent greater chance than a white of developing high blood pressure. And blacks under age 50 run six to seven times the risk of dying from hypertension-caused illnesses. High blood pressure among blacks also begins earlier in life and is more severe than among whites.

Heredity may be one reason for this racial difference. It is possible that the combination of genes leading to hypertension occurs more frequently in blacks than in whites.

Also possible is that the overall quality of health care afforded blacks is so much lower than that provided to whites that a greater percentage of the black population is "allowed" to develop hypertension.

Even if health-care variations account for some of the racial differences, it does not explain the fact that when blacks die from the results of hypertension, they succumb more often to strokes than to disease of the arteries supplying blood to the heart, the exact opposite of hypertensive whites.

Sex

Up to age 55, high blood pressure is less common among women than men. In the mid-50s both sexes have close to the same chance of developing the illness. And in later years, women are found to have high blood pressure more frequently than men. It is not known precisely why these differences exist.

Age

Most studies of blood-pressure changes show that hypertension increases with age. Some doctors maintain that this is probably due to the loss of the arteries' ability to stretch as the years go by.

Seldom, however, does blood pressure increase so dramatically after age 50 that hypertension can only then be diagnosed. Most instances of hypertension can be diagnosed by the age of 30 or 35, and often earlier, if appropriate tests are made.

Even among children and young adults, tendencies toward hypertension can be spotted by a physician aware of the normal blood-pressure levels for the ages of the patients involved. In general it is normal for blood pressure to increase slightly as children grow into their teenage years.

Among people diagnosed as mildly hypertensive, the incidence of stroke brought on by high blood pressure gradually increases with age, until in their 60s and 70s both men and women with untreated high blood pressure face strokes as a leading cause of disability and death.

3.

THE DANGERS OF HIGH BLOOD PRESSURE

- *High blood pressure is a silent killer*
- *It causes disabling illnesses, including:*
  - *stroke*
  - *kidney damage*
  - *congestive heart failure*
  - *atherosclerosis*
  - *angina pectoris*
  - *heart attack*
- *Many who have high blood pressure are not aware of it*
- *Most people don't know enough about high blood pressure*

Hypertension can lead to many serious health problems, from an enlarged heart that can no longer function efficiently, to burst blood vessels in the brain that can kill instantly. Your kidneys can be seriously damaged by hypertension if it is not controlled early, and your blood vessels can become badly blocked by atherosclerosis after only a few years of untreated hypertension.

We'll look at each of the major results of hypertension.

Strokes

EARLY WARNING SIGNS OF STROKE

Many people who have suffered a stroke were warned, usually months in advance, that the stroke was imminent. The warning came in the form of a temporary strokelike symptom called a "trans-ischemic attack," or TIA. Too often, unless their victims are alerted to them, TIAs are dismissed as unimportant. A TIA is caused by a temporary blockage of blood to part of the brain.

Some TIA signs:

• Dizziness lasting for a few minutes without apparent reason

• Numbness in the arms or legs, again without apparent reason (such as a sharp blow or other obvious injury)

• Tingling (pins-and-needles) in the limbs

• Temporary slurring of speech

IF YOU EXPERIENCE ANY OF THESE SYMPTOMS, CONSULT YOUR DOCTOR AT ONCE!

A stroke occurs when the blood supply to a portion of the brain is partly or totally cut off. Without enough blood, the brain cells starve to death. Strokes often affect the portions of the brain that control hand and arm movement, the sense of balance, or speech. When the cells that carry certain memories are destroyed, the memories are lost forever.

Many strokes are relatively minor. They might

cause a brief period of confusion or an episode of stumbling but will leave no lasting loss of ability.

Other strokes permanently paralyze much of the body.

Most strokes are caused by high blood pressure in two ways. *First:* Blood may burst through the wall of an artery already weakened by years of high blood pressure. The blood spills freely into the brain; millions of brain cells are suddenly deprived of the blood they need. A great deal of damage can be done by even a tiny stroke. *Second:* Untreated high blood pressure is a major contributor to hardening of the arteries. Fatty substances build up inside blood vessels. As these deposits increase, they can block blood flow to the brain.

In the United States and Canada, more than 400,000 people suffer strokes annually, and half of them die. One comprehensive study of the link between hypertension and strokes shows that people with high blood pressure are seven times more likely to have strokes than are those with normal blood pressure.

While strokes remain a major health problem worldwide and are significant causes of disability and death, an increasing number of people are avoiding this devastating illness due to better diagnosis of high blood pressure and increased acceptance of the many treatments available.

Congestive Heart Failure

Congestive heart failure occurs when the heart can no longer pump strongly enough to push blood into the body against the constant pressure of blood already filling the arteries and veins. It is, in effect, the result of a battle between systolic and diastolic blood pressures (systolic is the heart's pumping force; diastolic is the force from blood vessels).

As the heart vainly tries to pump, the walls of the heart stretch and become weaker and weaker, until they lose their elasticity and can no longer pump blood with adequate pressure.

CONGESTIVE HEART FAILURE WARNINGS

Congestive heart failure frequently causes edema, the buildup of fluids throughout the body, most often in the legs, and sometimes in the lungs.

Some symptoms of congestive heart failure to watch out for:

• *Persistent swollen ankles. If you press your finger against your ankle and the depressed area pushes back out immediately, it may be a sign of edema, especially if the swelling came on gradually (over a period of a few months), without extensive walking or standing, and it does not go away even after resting.*

• *Severe, persistent coughing, sometimes waking you up in the middle of the night, without a cause you can identify (such as heavy smoking). This may be a sign of fluid buildup in the lungs.*

• *Persistent shortness of breath without corresponding exercise.*

IF YOU EXPERIENCE ANY OF THESE SYMPTOMS, CONSULT YOUR DOCTOR AT ONCE!

Eventually, fluids that make up the blood start to fill the lungs, the veins, and other tissues of the abdomen and legs, creating the condition called edema. A collection of excess fluids in the lungs, termed pulmonary edema, can lead to death through suffocation.

Individuals who have untreated high blood pressure are four to six times more likely than others to develop congestive heart failure. Even if blood pressure is only a few points above normal, there is twice the chance of developing this ailment.

Hardening of the Arteries (Atherosclerosis)

Hardening of the arteries, which the medical profession calls atherosclerosis, is the result of fatty deposits building up in the arteries.

If the deposits are thick enough, they slow down the flow of blood; eventually, they may completely block the flow, causing a stroke (if blood to the brain is shut off) or a heart attack (if blood to the heart itself is blocked). A condition called angina pectoris—serious chest pains sometimes described as "crushing" pains—results from a blockage of the arteries that carry blood to the heart itself. These pains are the main warning sign that arteries may be blocked by atherosclerosis.

People who have high blood pressure develop atherosclerosis two decades earlier than those who have normal blood pressure.

Hypertensives have a 200 to 400 percent greater chance of having a heart attack caused by atherosclerosis that cuts off blood to part of the heart.

Kidney Damage

When arteries that supply blood to the kidneys become blocked, the kidneys can no longer efficiently clean waste materials out of the blood. Unless blood pressure is held down, the kidneys eventually fail.

In addition, since the kidneys produce a hormone that regulates blood pressure, lack of adequate blood to the kidneys further disrupts the blood-pressure-control system all over the body. There are no obvious early signs of kidney damage caused by high blood pressure, but in advanced cases the damage can range from changes in urinary frequency to total kidney failure.

Hypertension is the leading cause of kidney disease, which kills 60,000 Americans yearly.

4.

LIVING WITH HIGH BLOOD PRESSURE

- *You can lead a normal life with high blood pressure*
- *Continued blood pressure monitoring is essential*
- *Keeping in touch with your doctor is a matter of life and death*
- *Don't try to make too many changes at once in your lifestyle*
- *You—and only you—can affect your high blood pressure*

You are the only person who can control your high blood pressure.

Your doctor can diagnose the illness, prescribe medications, suggest changes in your lifestyle, and offer support to help you avoid the dangers of hypertension. But it is *you* who must take the prescribed medication, and *you* who might have to stick to a diet or get more exercise.

The underlying threat of high blood pressure stems from the fact that it doesn't hurt. Without a distinct pain or some other obvious symptom, the illness is not taken seriously by many of its victims.

They don't take their drugs as prescribed, they don't see their doctors regularly, they ignore their diets, and they fail to get enough exercise.

Other people fail to control their blood pressure because they try *too* hard. They attempt to go on a diet, to start exercising, to stop smoking, *and* to worry less about their jobs all at once. And when they are overwhelmed by the hard work involved in making so many changes, they give up on them all, even neglecting their medicine.

Yet another problem is that sometimes people don't give their drugs enough time to work, and stop taking them after only a few days when their blood pressure fails to respond. Some of the medications described in this book take several days, even weeks, to take effect and must be taken exactly as prescribed to work properly. Give them a chance.

It is equally dangerous to stop taking hypertension medications when blood pressure *does* drop, unless you are instructed to do so by your doctor. The drugs may have been the only reason for the drop, and blood pressure will rise again without them.

The most important thing you can do is to continue taking the drugs your doctor has prescribed. Before starting a diet or making some other major change in your life, get used to taking your medication on a regular basis. It is the cornerstone of successful hypertension treatment. If you experience unpleasant side effects, tell your doctor about them, but DON'T STOP TAKING THE DRUGS. Your physician may change the type of medication or its strength to ease any discomfort.

When you are accustomed to the medication and ready to begin a lifestyle change to help lower your blood pressure, discuss with your doctor what to try first. Perhaps exercise is more important for you than a diet, or learning to take it easy at work is more important than exercise. A step-by-step approach offers the greatest chance of success, and your doctor can help you decide which step to take first.

It is crucial that you continue to see your doctor regularly. Don't cancel an appointment just because you didn't lose as much weight as you wanted to lose or didn't jog as often as he suggested. With high blood pressure, your doctor's job is not to judge you, but to work as your partner in finding the best ways to keep down your blood pressure, ways that work for you.

Living with high blood pressure does not mean (except in the most severe, rare cases) that your life has to change dramatically. You'll be able to do all the things you've always enjoyed, although you may have to do some of them with a bit more moderation.

Even insurance companies recognize the advantages of continuing treatment. *The Journal of the American Medical Association* reports that most major medical insurance firms across the country offer normal rates to those with high blood pressure, *as long as the hypertension treatment continues successfully.*

If you stick to your treatment plan, your hypertension will be brought under control. If for some reason you stop treatment, don't waste your energy feeling guilty about it; instead, start the treatment again, trying to avoid the circumstances that made you stop the first time.

Don't let high blood pressure win!

5.

YOUR TREATMENT AND YOU

- *High blood pressure can be treated*
- *You determine the effectiveness of the treatment*
- *Drugs can control high blood pressure*
- *Lifestyle changes can help lower blood pressure*
- *Nondrug treatments work, too*

Once your high blood pressure has been diagnosed, a large part of your treatment is in your hands. High blood pressure is unlike most other illnesses. Usually, you will visit a doctor when you experience distinct symptoms—a cough, a pain, perhaps a cut or a burn. Not so with hypertension. Instead, you are asked to accept the doctor's word that you are ill, even though you have no symptoms.

High-blood-pressure treatment can involve medications, diet, and/or exercise. You may be urged to take drugs—for the rest of your life, perhaps—without ever having actually "experienced" any symptoms of the illness. Complete descriptions of drugs prescribed today, including their sometimes bothersome side effects, begin on p. 65.

Most of these medicines produce no adverse side effects; only about 15 percent of hypertension patients report any problems with the drugs their doctors prescribe.

If you do encounter unpleasant side effects from a drug prescribed for you, tell your doctor about them. Most likely the dosage can be reduced, or a substitute medication or combination of drugs can be prescribed as a replacement.

Despite side effects, it is vitally important to your health—and your life—that you take the medicine as prescribed. Most side effects are due to the fact that, in many cases, the body requires weeks or months to grow accustomed to new medication.

If your physician suggests you begin a diet and/or exercise program as part of your treatment, discuss with him how likely you are to continue such a program. It's possible that the doctor will suggest alternatives if a diet or exercise program is too difficult for you to undertake.

QUESTIONS AND ANSWERS ABOUT HIGH BLOOD PRESSURE

Q. How do I know whether I have high blood pressure?

A. You should trust only a doctor, trained medical worker, or yourself (after proper instruction) to accurately record your blood pressure. A doctor should diagnose hypertension only after several blood-pressure readings are taken.

Q. Can I avoid taking medication?

A. If your blood pressure is only slightly above normal, you may be able to lower it to safe levels through diet, exercise, and/or training to reduce the effects of stress. Ask your doctor about these alternatives. If your blood pressure is seriously elevated, you will without doubt have to take drugs.

Q. If my blood pressure goes down, can I stop the drugs?

A. If your blood pressure was only a little higher than normal, and you lost weight or exercised substantially since hypertension was diagnosed, your doctor may be willing to stop the drugs to determine whether blood pressure can be controlled without them. Do not stop taking the medications without consulting your doctor.

Q. My doctor makes me take several different pills. Why can't I take just one a day?

A. High blood pressure treatment may require a combination of very different drug groups. If you have trouble keeping track of the various pills your doctor prescribed, ask him about pills that combine several drugs in a single dose. The medications you require may not be available in combination pills, or may be available in doses your doctor does not recommend for you.

Q. My doctor has changed my medications several times. Why can't he get the prescription right?

A. Everyone responds a little differently to hypertension medications. Your doctor is probably trying to find the precise drug, or combination of drugs, that works best for you and reduces side effects as much as possible.

Q. I have some side effects from the high blood pressure medication, but my doctor won't try different drugs. What can I do?

A. It is the doctor's responsibility to search for the drugs that best meet your medical needs. If you are not satisfied with his choices, and he cannot offer satisfactory reasons for selecting the drugs he prescribed, your alternative is to find another doctor who is more interested in your health care. Ask your friends and family members for recommendations. Hypertension is a common enough illness that several people you know may well be undergoing treatment right now and can suggest another doctor.

Q. My friend's medicine really lowered her blood pressure. Can I try some of it?

A. NO! You may respond completely differently from your friend, and trying that medication could be extremely dangerous to you. You should never use someone else's prescription drugs.

Q. TV and newspaper ads for private clinics sometimes say they can cure hypertension without drugs. Why can't my doctor?

A. When blood pressure is just a little bit high, weight loss and exercise may be enough to reduce it to normal levels. You should ask your doctor if your blood pressure might be reduced this way, or whether it is so high that drugs are essential.

Q. **My father was on a low-salt diet for hypertension, but my doctor says I shouldn't bother with diet foods or low-salt products. Who's right?**

A. Many physicians believe the immediate goal is to reduce the blood pressure, and drugs usually do that faster than dietary changes. With mild hypertension, a diet can eventually take the place of medications in some cases. There is much controversy over whether reducing salt will help reduce high blood pressure, but most doctors—to "play it safe"—suggest that their hypertensive patients cut down on salt.

Alternative Treatments

While most physicians prefer to treat all but the mildest cases of hypertension with drugs, nontraditional treatments are available to those who wish to avoid the possible side effects of medications or for some other reason are inclined to try alternative methods of lowering blood pressure.

Most of these treatment styles deal with stress, a common hypertension risk factor. Some treatments lower the level of stress; others change the way you deal with stressful situations. Each method has proponents ready to assure you that the treatments will work well to lower your blood pressure. Some alternative treatment methods are available through stress clinics, advertised in newspapers and magazines, or taught in night classes at colleges. An increasing number of physicians are learning more about some of the methods and how their patients can take advantage of them.

One clinic that offers alternative treatments even advertises a money-back guarantee if, after several weeks of nondrug therapy, a patient's blood pressure is not lowered.

The treatments are based primarily on what is now called the "relaxation response."

Normally, when confronted with a stressful situation, a "fight or flight" response is automatic; that is, you must either flee the stress or vigorously fight its cause. If you can be taught to face a stressful situation by relaxing instead, your blood pressure is unlikely to rise dangerously.

Some methods for consciously controlling the body's response to stress, like yoga and Zen Buddhism, have been known in Eastern countries for centuries. Others are based on modern technology.

Yoga

In India, people have been seeking the road to peace of mind, and deeper insights into the nature of reality, for hundreds—perhaps thousands—of years. Teachers, or yogis, emerged who had worked out systems of meditation said to enable people to better comprehend the self and to find freedom, happiness, and tranquility with the universe.

One of the systems the yogis teach is "hatha" yoga, which uses postures and exercises (asanas), breath control (pranayama), and meditation (dhyana) to elicit relaxation. Some of the breathing exercises are reputed to lower blood pressure.

Of the various nontraditional methods of treating hypertension, yoga holds the greatest promise.

It is the best studied, although much research remains to be conducted before it becomes widely accepted by the Western medical community as an alternative to drug therapy.

Yoga exercises should always be learned under the guidance of a trained, qualified teacher.

Zen Buddhism

The meditative techniques of ancient Zen Buddhism were perfected in Japan and are based on even older Chinese relaxation methods. Meditation involves concentrating on breathing and performing other physical and mental exercises. Zen Buddhism, in this regard, can help lower blood pressure much the way yoga does.

Transcendental Meditation [TM]

Transcendental meditation can be learned by anyone in just a few hours. Relaxation is brought about by the individual getting comfortable (perhaps in an easy chair), breathing regularly, closing the eyes, and repeating—at first aloud, then silently—a single word, most often a "mantra," which is usually a word-sound from the Sanskrit language.

Progressive Muscle Relaxation [PMR]

Progressive muscle relaxation attempts to control stress through rhythmic tightening and relaxing of various muscles. It can be performed in virtually any position—sitting, lying down, standing—and can be directed toward any group of muscles. PMR can be used by a business executive even during a meeting or by a schoolteacher during class.

Biofeedback

In biofeedback, a mechanical or electrical device wired to the body, such as a buzzer or a light, lets the subject know when a desired physical or mental state is reached.

With hypertension, a buzzer might sound whenever blood pressure is above a predetermined level. The biofeedback subject tries various relaxation methods until the buzzer stops, and then attempts to keep the buzzer from sounding again.

This method can help train some individuals to control otherwise involuntary physical responses to stress.

Hypnosis

Hypnosis may be helpful for some people by encouraging their cooperation in programs to reduce their hypertension risk—for example, by increasing confidence in their ability to lose weight or to exercise more regularly. However, it is questionable whether hypnosis causes a direct reduction in blood pressure.

Traditional Treatments

In addition to prescribing medications to help control your high blood pressure, your doctor may encourage you to:

- Begin a diet if you are overweight
- Exercise more
- Change other eating habits if necessary
- Avoid stressful situations

In the following pages, we'll talk about each of these suggestions your doctor might make.

Losing Weight

If you are too heavy for your height and build, your doctor will most likely suggest that you lose weight in order to reduce your blood pressure.

Men and women, once they reach adulthood, gradually require less food. The decline in nutrition requirement is not much in one year, but over two decades it can make a world of difference. Yet, many adults eat the same amount of food at age 40 as they did at 20. And they wonder why they gain weight.

As we have seen, overweight tends to increase blood pressure. A lower-calorie diet may be necessary. Recently, weight tables were updated by the Metropolitan Life Insurance Company to reflect new research into the weight levels beyond which health may be endangered.

To lose weight successfully, there is no need to go on any crash or fad diet. Instead, begin by checking your eating habits against a good food guide to make sure you are getting proper nutrition.

You will probably find your diet needs some adjustment to include more fiber and less salt, cholesterol, sugar, and other high-calorie foods. Then, experiment with the portions a bit. Cut down your normal portions, if possible by as much as half.

To establish your current eating habits, you may want to carry a small notebook and record every bit of food and drink you consume for three days—a weekend and one weekday.

Then purchase a pocket calorie counter (at your local pharmacy, supermarket, or bookstore) and write down how many calories you consumed each day. Probably you'll find about five hundred calories you can eliminate without too much trouble.

Above all, keep in mind that since you put on

IDEAL WEIGHT (LBS.)

MEN

HEIGHT	SMALL	BODY FRAME SIZE MEDIUM	LARGE
5' 2"	125–134	131–141	138–150
5' 3"	130–136	133–143	140–153
5' 4"	132–138	135–145	142–156
5' 5"	134–140	137–148	144–160
5' 6"	136–142	139–151	146–164
5' 7"	138–145	142–154	149–168
5' 8"	140–148	145–157	152–172
5' 9"	142–151	148–160	155–176
5'10"	144–154	151–163	158–180
5'11"	146–157	154–166	161–184
6' 0"	149–160	157–170	164–188
6' 1"	152–164	160–174	168–192
6' 2"	156–168	164–178	172–197
6' 3"	158–172	167–182	176–202
6' 4"	162–176	171–187	181–207

WOMEN

4'10"	102–111	109–121	118–131
4'11"	103–113	111–123	120–134
5'0"	104–115	113–126	122–137
5'1"	106–118	115–129	125–140
5'2"	108–121	118–132	128–143
5'3"	111–124	121–135	131–147
5'4"	114–127	124–138	134–151
5'5"	117–130	127–141	137–155
5'6"	120–133	130–144	140–159
5'7"	123–136	133–147	143–163
5'8"	126–139	136–150	146–167
5'9"	129–142	139–153	149–170
5'10"	132–145	142–156	152–173
5'11"	135–148	145–159	155–176
6'0"	138–151	148–162	158–179

Chart is for people aged 25–59, in shoes and wearing five pounds of indoor clothing for men, three pounds for women.

the weight gradually, it is best to lose it gradually, too. The slow loss comes with a change in eating habits, and only this change will enable you to keep your weight down permanently.

Fad diets can help you lose weight in a hurry, but you will surely put it back on just as quickly.

The reason most diets fail is twofold. People demand from themselves diet adjustments that, in the long run, they cannot possibly maintain; and they expect the diets drastically to change their lives. For instance, the dieter is disappointed when the dream man or woman fails to materialize. When change doesn't occur, they return to their old eating habits and gain back the weight.

For your diet to be successful, you must be realistic about it. The goal of a diet is simply to lose weight, and the loss of weight may help you reduce your blood pressure. It should certainly help you feel better.

Exercise

Some exercise will almost certainly be part of your doctor's prescribed hypertension treatment.

Exercise can do much more than help you lose weight. It can improve your overall outlook and promote relaxation. Exercise gives you a chance to release emotions that would otherwise be turned inward, to your detriment. Some authorities even believe that exercise can by itself lower the diastolic pressure by opening small blood vessels deep within the muscles.

There is one cardinal rule underlying all exercise: if you've been leading a sedentary life, return to activity gradually and cautiously. There is no reason why you cannot achieve peak fitness for your age at any time in your life, but the older you get, the more cautious you have to be at the start.

Talk to your doctor about how strenuously you should exercise at first and how you can tell when you're overdoing it as you progress with your exercise program.

In general, the exercises that have the greatest potential for lowering your blood pressure are those that stretch your muscles rhythmically, rather than those that cause you to exert yourself to excess for brief periods. Lifting weights is a poor exercise for hypertensives; running and swimming are much better ones.

A good way to start an exercise program is by walking briskly. A "brisk" pace is about 100–130 steps per minute. Simple devices are available at many sporting-goods stores to record the number of paces you take per minute. For the first five minutes of each walk, start off slowly, then gradually pick up your pace until you are walking briskly.

Try not to break your stride. Good exercise is continuous. Each walk should last at least thirty minutes, but be sure to establish a pace and time limit you're comfortable with, and work up from there.

To judge your own limit, stop exercising when you reach the point of breathlessness or are unable to talk easily. A good schedule is to walk three or four times weekly, at least thirty minutes per walk. But DON'T OVERDO IT; work your way up to that schedule slowly.

Stress

Your physician might urge you to "take life a bit easier" or "learn to enjoy yourself more." What he means is: reduce stress.

According to Hans Selye, the researcher who pioneered modern stress research, stress is basically "the rate of wear and tear within the body." It becomes harmful when the rate is unnecessarily great, a situation that can be called "negative stress." With negative stress, the body is continually in an "alarm state," during which muscles are tense, geared up for an emergency.

There is, on the other hand, "positive stress," which actually enhances life and spurs a person on to greater productivity and satisfaction. Unfortunately, the stress encountered by most people is

---

HOW TO HANDLE STRESS

Besides the approaches to stress already discussed as part of the nontraditional treatments for hypertension (see p. 40), the National Association of Mental Health outlines other ways to deal with stress:

• **Let It Out.** When something worries you, don't bottle it up. Confide your problem to some level-headed individual you can trust: a family member, friend, doctor, clergyman, or teacher. Or, if you don't know anyone who wants to hear your problem, try one of the hotlines in your city or county.

• **Change Your Goals.** Determine whether your personal and career goals are realistic. Talk them over with someone. Are you biting off more than you can chew? Taking on too much responsibility? Don't be afraid to revise your goals to make them more realistic.

• **Work on Your Attitude.** Consider which irritants bother you. Are they really serious, or are they minor? Try to convince yourself that the minor irritants are not worth the trouble of worrying about.

negative and must be brought under control.

People are not affected adversely by stress until the stress becomes negative; that is, when they begin to perceive the stress as bothersome.

Each individual's perception of stress determines whether it is positive or negative, but for most people stress becomes negative when they feel they are losing control over their own actions and when their self-image diminishes.

• **Work It Off.** *Physical activity—a long walk, tennis, carpentry, a hobby—will leave you better prepared to deal with your stress in a calm and intelligent way. It helps put you back in control.*

• **Rehearse Stressful Events.** *When you anticipate being thrown into a possibly stressful event, think through in advance what might happen, and consider responses you might make. Run them through your mind like a play, and script things so you come out all right.*

• **Manage Your Time.** *Plan in advance; fill up only half of your day with scheduled events. Don't set impossible time schedules for meetings, shopping, or even visiting friends. Keep a calendar or pocket schedule, and make sure it has lots of open time.*

• **One Thing at a Time.** *Try to convince yourself that it doesn't help to worry about your afternoon meeting when you're still in your morning meeting. Handle the first task first, then move on to the next.*

• **Avoid Certain Situations.** *If you get particularly tense in traffic jams, say, try to avoid them by changing your travel schedule whenever possible.*

Smoking

Although the tie between smoking and hypertension is unclear, those who have high blood pressure and who also smoke are known to run a dramatically increased risk of stroke. While smoking does not appear to cause high blood pressure, it does cause harm, and it may weaken the body sufficiently to make hypertension more likely. To stop smoking will be an important recommendation from your doctor.

Salt

A decade ago, physicians almost always suggested that hypertensive patients cut their salt intake. Although recent studies indicate that a reduction in salt does little to reduce blood pressure, doctors continue to urge their patients to cut down on salt, in the belief that caution in the face of controversy is the best route to follow.

6.

HIGH BLOOD PRESSURE DRUG TREATMENTS

- *Many types of medications can reduce blood pressure*
- *Some drugs decrease the body's fluid content*
- *Others dilate blood vessels*
- *Some affect the nervous system*
- *Drug combinations are often prescribed*

Dozens of drugs are commonly prescribed for high blood pressure. Today's array of hypertension drugs is much broader than it was just a few years ago. And, after decades of research, they are becoming increasingly safer.

While mild high blood pressure can often be controlled by exercise, diet, or lifestyle changes alone, many physicians will still prescribe drugs because some of their patients have difficulty in losing weight or maintaining an exercise program.

Some hypertension medications decrease the fluid content of the blood. Others have an impact on the nervous system, which ultimately controls everything the heart and blood vessels do. Still others cause the muscles of the blood vessels themselves to dilate, thus allowing the blood to flow under less pressure.

Once high blood pressure is diagnosed, most doctors follow one of two courses of drug treatment.

Course A

Depending on an individual's particular circumstances, including his overall state of health and previous experience with drugs, the physician may first try to control hypertension with a diuretic, which reduces the salt and fluid content of the body and the blood. If blood pressure does not drop sufficiently, a beta blocker may be added to slow down the heartbeat.

If the hypertension remains uncontrolled, a vasodilator, which opens the blood vessels wider, may be added to the drug-treatment schedule. If the combination of three medications is ineffective, a drug that acts on the nervous system may be added.

Course B

A few cases of high blood pressure respond better to a treatment plan that begins with a beta blocker, rather than a diuretic, which may still be added if the beta blocker alone does not control the hypertension. The balance of the drug schedule—adding a vasodilator, then a drug that acts on the nervous system, if the more-limited therapy does not work well enough—remains the same.

"Stepped Care" Drug Treatment

Physicians call this method of beginning treatment with the mildest drugs possible, and progressing to more powerful drugs only if required, a "stepped care" program. It can best be understood in the form of a diagram, with the initial stages of drug treatment starting at the bottom:

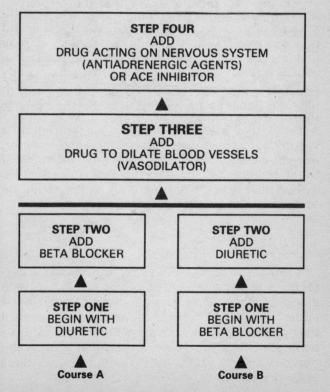

The drugs used for each step of hypertension treatment are described in detail in the following section.

New drugs to control hypertension are sometimes developed that do not fall within traditional courses of treatment. For example, a new class of drugs called indolines has properties of both vasodilators and diuretics, and is prescribed both alone and in combination with other medications.

Vital to the success of any drug-treatment schedule is the relationship between patient and doctor. The patient should be aware that the prescribed drugs may require a few changes in dosage and type to reduce side effects, and that sometimes the doctor needs weeks, or even months, to find the right medication or combination of medications. The doctor, meanwhile, must pay attention to the patient's concerns about side effects and recognize the patient's limitations if a diet or exercise program is recommended.

II
The Most Commonly Prescribed High Blood Pressure Drugs in the United States, Generic and Brand Names, with Complete Descriptions of Drugs and Their Effects

1.

GENERAL INFORMATION ABOUT DRUG TYPES

Following is general information about the different types of drugs commonly used to treat high blood pressure. Specific information about your drug can be found in the next section, where drugs are listed alphabetically by their generic names. If you have trouble locating your drug, please consult the index (p. 187).

Diuretics

Thiazide Diuretics

Bendroflumethiazide (see p. 77)
Benzthiazide (see p. 80)
Chlorothiazide (see p. 88)
Cyclothiazide (see p. 95)
Hydrochlorothiazide (see p. 116)
Hydroflumethiazide (see p. 119)
Methyclothiazide (see p. 126)
Polythiazide (see p. 148)
Quinethazone (see p. 158)
Trichlormethiazide (see p. 175)

Thiazidelike Diuretics

Chlorthalidone (see p. 91)
Metolazone (see p. 132)

Loop Diuretics

Bumetanide (see p. 83)
Ethacrynic Acid (see p. 103)
Furosemide (see p. 105)

Potassium-Sparing Diuretics

Amiloride Hydrochloride (see p. 72)
Spironolactone (see p. 168)
Triamterene (see p. 173)

Since the late 1950s, diuretics—or "water pills"—have been the standard first-line drug therapy for high blood pressure. In many cases, diuretics alone control mild or moderate hypertension, and they are usually the first drug doctors prescribe for hypertensive patients.

Diuretics help to lower blood pressure by reducing the amount of liquid in the blood. By decreasing the amount of fluid that must be handled by your circulatory system, pressure inside your blood vessels goes down. Diuretics reduce fluids by inhibiting the body's ability to absorb sodium and water, which are then eliminated from the body with urine. The result is the most common side effect of diuretics: an increase in the frequency of urination and the volume of urine.

Diuretics used to treat hypertension are divided into groups according to their chemical structures and to where they act in the kidneys.

Thiazide diuretics often initiate the drug treatment program. If they fail to control blood pressure, then the more potent *loop diuretics* may be tried.

The major drawback to these diuretics is their potential for causing electrolyte or mineral imbalances, such as decreased potassium and bicarbonate levels. If you take diuretics, pay special attention to the warning signs for electrolyte imbalance discussed under your drug's *Possible Side Effects* section.

If potassium loss becomes a problem for you, your doctor may prescribe *potassium-sparing diuretics* such as spironolactone or triamterene, which do not cause significant potassium loss. However, they may not be as effective as other diuretics. Your doctor may also suggest a potassium supplement (see p. 150) or foods rich in potassium (bananas, melons, citrus fruits, tomatoes).

Or, your doctor may prescribe a diuretic-combination drug, in which one ingredient counteracts the potassium loss caused by the diuretic.

Diuretic Combinations

Aldactazide (see p. 65)
Aldoril (see p. 68)
Dyazide (see p. 100)
Inderide (see p. 124)
Moduretic (see p. 139)
Ser-Ap-Es (see p. 166)

These combination drugs, with their fixed dosage levels, are not used for the initial treatment of hypertension. Rather, they are used when there is a need to add another drug, and when you desire the convenience of taking only one pill. You should always remember that the treatment of hypertension is not static—the type of medications and the dosage amounts involved may change, so it is important that you remain under your doctor's care to insure that you are getting exactly what you need to treat your condition.

Some other combination brand-name antihypertensives (and their ingredients) are:

Brand Name	Ingredients
Apresazide	Hydralazine Hydrochloride (see p. 114)
	Hydrochlorothiazide (see p. 116)
Combipres	Chlorthalidone (see p. 91)
	Clonidine Hydrochloride (see p. 93)
Demi-Regroton	Chlorthalidone (see p. 91)
	Reserpine (see p. 163)
Diupres	Chlorothiazide (see p. 88)
	Reserpine (see p. 163)
Enduronyl	Deserpidine (see p. 98)
	Methyclothiazide (see p. 126)
Esimil	Guanethidine Sulfate (see p. 112)
	Hydrochlorothiazide (see p. 116)
Hydropres	Hydrochlorothiazide (see p. 116)
	Reserpine (see p. 163)
Regroton	Chlorthalidone (see p. 91)
	Reserpine (see p. 163)
Salutensin	Hydroflumethiazide (see p. 119)
	Reserpine (see p. 163)
Serpasil-Apresoline	Reserpine (see p. 163)
	Hydralazine Hydrochloride (see p. 114)

Since these drugs are combinations of at least two generic drugs, it is extremely important that you refer to the descriptions of the generic ingredients for information regarding cautions and warnings, side effects, adverse effects, and drug interactions that may affect you when taking the combination drug.

Beta Blockers

Atenolol (see p. 74)
Metoprolol Tartrate (see p. 134)
Nadolol (see p. 142)
Pindolol (see p. 145)
Propranolol Hydrochloride (see p. 155)
Timolol Maleate (see p. 170)

Beta blockers are a relatively new class of drugs. Propranolol hydrochloride—the first beta blocker—was introduced in 1965. A new beta blocker—labetalol—was recently approved by the Federal government, and may soon become widely prescribed because, in clinical trials, it appears to work for some people who do not respond well to other drugs. Labetalol will be sold under the brand names Normodyne and Trandate. Exactly how these drugs reduce blood pressure is not yet known. It is thought that they block the effect of naturally occurring stimulants (i.e. norepinephrine) on the "beta" receptors found in the heart and in some blood vessels. They produce several important changes in body functions: slow the heartbeat, reduce the amount of blood pumped by the heart, cause dilation of some major blood vessels, and offset some of the usual physiological effects of natural body stimulants. This ultimately results in lowered blood pressure. In addition, beta blockers may be used to treat a variety of conditions including abnormal heart rhythms, angina, glaucoma, hyperthyroid disease, and migraines.

Beta blockers can be prescribed as the first drug in the treatment of hypertension, or when a diuretic alone has failed to lower blood pressure. They may be prescribed alone or in combination with other antihypertensive medications.

Vasodilators

Hydralazine Hydrochloride (see p. 114)
Minoxidil (see p. 137)
Prazosin Hydrochloride (see p. 153)

Vasodilators reduce blood pressure by directly relaxing the muscles responsible for tightening blood vessels, thus making it easier for the heart to pump blood, and thereby lowering blood pressure. These drugs are closely related to the peripherally acting antiadrenergic agents (i.e., clonidine and methyldopa). In fact, prazosin hydrochloride is often considered an antiadrenergic agent.

As a rule, vasodilators are not prescribed unless other drug treatments have failed to lower blood pressure. They are almost always prescribed in combination with other antihypertensive medications such as diuretics or beta blockers.

In general, vasodilators may be used to treat a variety of conditions ranging from angina to Alzheimer's disease. However, the vasodilators listed in this section are used primarily to treat hypertension.

Antiadrenergic Agents

Clonidine Hydrochloride (see p. 93)
Guanabenz Acetate (see p. 108)
Guanadrel Sulfate (see p. 110)
Guanethidine Sulfate (see p. 112)
Methyldopa (see p. 129)

These drugs are classified as antiadrenergic agents because they inhibit adrenergic reactions. (*Adrenergic* is the term for motor nerves that use epinephrine or norepinephrine to transmit the impulses believed to be responsible for increased blood pressure.) When these adrenergic reactions are blocked, your blood pressure decreases.

Usually, these drugs are prescribed when diuretics alone have failed to lower blood pressure. These antiadrenergic agents may be prescribed by themselves, but they are frequently prescribed together with other antihypertensive medications.

Rauwolfia Derivatives

Alseroxylon (see p. 72)
Deserpidine (see p. 110)
Rescinnamine (see p. 183)
Reserpine (see p. 163)
Whole Root Rauwolfia (see p. 205)

Rauwolfia-derivative drugs are considered antiadrenergic agents (see p. 63)—a group of antihypertensive medications that appear to lower blood pressure through their ability to decrease resistance within the blood vessels, thereby making it easier for the heart to pump blood.

These drugs are not usually used for the initial treatment of hypertension, but are generally prescribed only after diuretic drugs have failed to work adequately. These drugs are increasingly being supplanted by more potent drugs but remain available for the treatment of hypertension. Many of them are also prescribed as antipsychotic medications.

ACE Inhibitors

Captopril (see p. 86)

This drug is the first member of a new class of drugs (ACE inhibitors) that prevent the conversion of a potent hormone called angiotensin I-converting enzyme (ACE). This directly affects the production of other hormones and enzymes that participate in the regulation of blood pressure. The effect is to lower blood pressure quickly, within 1 to 1½ hours after taking the medicine.

Captopril can cause serious side effects and should be used only by those who have not responded to other antihypertensive medications.

Indolines

Indapamide (see p. 122)

Indapamide is the first representative of a new class of drugs called indolines. Indapamide combines many of the properties found in vasodilators and diuretics. It appears to work by relaxing the muscles responsible for tightening blood vessels, thus making it easier for the heart to pump blood, and thereby lowering blood pressure. In addition, this drug works as a diuretic by decreasing the amount of liquid that must be pumped through your blood vessels, which again results in lower blood pressure. Indapamide may be prescribed by itself or in combination with other antihypertensive medications.

MAO Inhibitors

Drugs known as MAO inhibitors, such as pargyline hydrochloride (Eutonyl), are rarely, but sometimes, prescribed for hypertension. If you are taking an MAO inhibitor, please consult your doctor for more information.

2.

DRUG PROFILES

Brand Name
Aldactazide

Ingredients

Hydrochlorothiazide
Spironolactone

Other Brand Names

Alazide
Spiractazide
Spironazide
Spironolactone with Hydrochlorothiazide
Spirozide

Type of Drug

Antihypertensive medication combining a thiazide diuretic (hydrochlorothiazide) with a potassium-sparing diuretic (spironolactone).

Prescribed for

The treatment of hypertension when it is necessary to counteract the potassium loss caused by
diuretics.

Cautions and Warnings

Do not take Aldactazide if you have severe kidney
disease, if you may be allergic to this drug or
to any sulfa drug, or if you have a history of allergy or bronchial asthma. Aldactazide may be used
to treat specific conditions in pregnant women,
but the decision by pregnant women to use this
medication should be weighed carefully because
the drug may cross the placental barrier and pass
into the blood of the unborn child. Aldactazide
may appear in the breast milk of nursing mothers.
Do not take any potassium supplements together
with Aldactazide unless specifically directed to do
so by your doctor.

This drug may cause drowsiness or sleepiness.
Do not drive or operate machinery. Call your doctor if you develop muscle or stomach cramps;
dizziness; nausea; diarrhea; unusual thirst; headache; rash; voice changes; breast enlargement;
unusual menstrual periods. This drug may be taken
with food to reduce stomach upset.

Possible Side Effects

Drowsiness; lethargy; headache; stomach upset;
cramping and diarrhea; rash; mental confusion;
fever; feeling of ill health; enlargement of the
breasts; inability to achieve or maintain erection
(in males); irregular menstrual cycles or deepening of the voice (in females).

Possible Adverse Effects

Loss of appetite; headache; tingling in the toes and fingers; restlessness; anemia or other effects on components of the blood; unusual sensitivity to sunlight; dizziness when rising quickly from a sitting position. Aldactazide can also produce muscle spasms; gout; weakness, and blurred vision.

Drug Interactions

Aldactazide may make the action of other blood-pressure-lowering drugs more effective. This is almost always a beneficial action, but your doctor may want to lower your dosage of the other antihypertensive drug.

The possibility of developing imbalances in body fluids and electrolytes is increased if you take other medications—such as digitalis and adrenal corticosteroids—while you are taking Aldactazide.

If you are taking an oral antidiabetic drug and begin taking Aldactazide, the antidiabetic dose may have to be altered.

Lithium carbonate should not be taken with Aldactazide because the combination may increase the risk of lithium toxicity.

Avoid over-the-counter cough, cold, or allergy remedies containing stimulant drugs that can aggravate your high blood pressure.

Aldactazide may interfere with the oral blood-thinning drugs (such as warfarin) by making the blood more concentrated (thicker).

Usual Dose

2 to 4 tablets daily, adjusted by your doctor until the desired therapeutic effect is achieved.

Overdosage

Symptoms are confusion, dizziness, nausea,

lethargy, coma. If you think you are experiencing an overdose, contact your doctor immediately, or go to a hospital emergency room. ALWAYS bring the medicine bottle with you.

Brand Name
Aldoril

Ingredients

Hydrochlorothiazide
Methyldopa

Type of Drug

Antihypertensive medication combining a diuretic (hydrochlorothiazide) with an antiadrenergic agent (methyldopa).

Prescribed for

The treatment of hypertension when the initial diuretic treatment does not provide satisfactory results.

Cautions and Warnings

Do not take Aldoril if you are allergic to either of its ingredients, if you have any liver diseases such as hepatitis or active cirrhosis, or if previous therapy with methyldopa has been associated with signs of liver reaction (jaundice or unexplained fever).

Aldoril will pass into the unborn child and can be found in mother's milk. Pregnant women should use this drugs only if it is absolutely necessary. Women taking Aldoril should not breast-feed their infants.

Aldoril may cause temporary mild sedation. Contact your doctor if your normal urine output is lessening or you are less hungry or are nauseated.

Be aware that Aldoril can cause orthostatic hypotension (dizziness when rising from a sitting or lying position). Alcohol will worsen this effect, so avoid alcohol at the beginning of Aldoril therapy.

You may take Aldoril with food to reduce upset stomach. Call your doctor if you develop muscle weakness, cramps, nausea, dizziness, fever, or tiredness.

Possible Side Effects

Loss of appetite; stomach upset; nausea; vomiting; cramps; diarrhea; constipation; dizziness; headache; tingling in the extremities; restlessness; chest pains; abnormal heart rhythms; drowsiness during the first few days of therapy.

Possible Adverse Effects

Aldoril can cause abnormal liver function in the first 2 to 3 months of therapy. Watch for jaundice (yellowing of the skin or whites of the eyes), with or without fever. If you are taking Aldoril for the first time, be sure your doctor checks your liver function, particularly during the first 6 to 12 weeks of therapy. If fever or jaundice appears, notify your doctor immediately. Other adverse effects: stuffy nose; breast enlargement; lactation (in females); impotence or decreased sex drive; mild arthritis; skin reactions such as mild eczema; stomach gas; dry mouth; sore or black tongue; fever.

Drug Interactions

Interaction with digitalis or quinidine can result in the development of abnormal heart rhythms.

Interaction with lithium products can lead to lithium toxicity unless appropriate dose adjustments are made.

Do not use over-the-counter cough, cold, or allergy remedies containing stimulant drugs that may raise your blood pressure. If you are not sure which over-the-counter drugs are safe for you, ask your doctor or pharmacist.

Usual Dose

Individualized to suit your needs.

Overdosage

Symptoms are confusion, dizziness, nausea, lethargy, coma. If you think you are experiencing an overdose, contact your doctor immediately, or go to a hospital emergency room. ALWAYS bring the medicine bottle with you.

Generic Name
Alseroxylon

Brand Name

Rauwiloid

Type of Drug

Antiadrenergic agent

Prescribed for

The treatment of hypertension—either alone or with other antihypertensive medications.

Cautions and Warnings

Do not stop taking alseroxylon unless directed to do so by your doctor.

Use with extreme caution if you suffer from depression, since alseroxylon may induce severe depression that may persist for several months after you stop taking it. Notify your doctor if you experience any changes in mood or sleep habits, or continual severe stomach pain.

Avoid cough, cold, or allergy medications except when they are approved by your doctor or pharmacist.

If dizziness occurs, avoid suddenly rising from a sitting or reclining position.

Pregnant women should use alseroxylon only when the potential benefits clearly outweigh the unknown potential hazards to the fetus.

Mothers should not breast-feed when taking alseroxylon.

Use alseroxylon with caution if you suffer from kidney or liver disease or have a history of peptic ulcers, ulcerative colitis, or gallstones.

This product may contain tartrazine, a substance found to cause allergic reactions, especially in people allergic to aspirin.

Possible Side Effects

Stuffy nose; dry mouth; dizziness; headache; breathing difficulties; impotence or decreased sex drive; muscle aches; weight gain; breast enlargement; lactation (in females).

Possible Adverse Effects

Nausea; vomiting; loss of appetite; diarrhea; stomach bleeding; chest pain; abnormal heart rhythms; swelling of hands or feet; depression;

fainting; involuntary movements or twitching of the head and neck.

Drug Interactions

Digitalis and quinidine, when used with alseroxylon, may cause abnormal heart rhythms.

MAO inhibitors should be avoided or used with extreme caution.

Alseroxylon, when used with beta blockers, may result in extreme low blood pressure manifested by fainting, vertigo, or dizziness when suddenly rising from a sitting or reclining position.

Usual Dose

Initial dose: 2 to 4 mg. daily.
Maintenance dose: 2 mg. daily.

Overdosage

Symptoms are changes in consciousness ranging from dizziness to coma; diarrhea; difficulty in breathing; slow heartbeat; flushing of the skin; pupil constriction. If you think you are experiencing an overdose, contact your doctor immediately, or go to a hospital emergency room. ALWAYS bring the medicine bottle with you.

Generic Name
Amiloride Hydrochloride

Brand Name

Midamor

Type of Drug

Potassium-sparing diuretic

Prescribed for

The treatment of hypertension when it is important to avoid the potassium loss caused by other diuretics. Amiloride hydrochloride is almost always prescribed in combination with other diuretics.

Cautions and Warnings

Use amiloride hydrochloride with extreme caution if you suffer from kidney or liver disease.

Do not take other potassium-sparing drugs (i.e., spironolactone or triamterene) while taking amiloride hydrochloride.

Avoid other forms of potassium supplements or a potassium-rich diet (i.e., bananas, citrus fruits, melons, tomatoes) unless your doctor specifically instructs you to increase your potassium intake while taking amiloride hydrochloride.

Diabetics should avoid using amiloride hydrochloride.

Pregnant women should use this drug only when the potential benefits clearly outweigh the unknown potential hazards to the fetus. The safety for nursing mothers using amiloride hydrochloride has not been established.

Amiloride hydrochloride may cause dizziness, headache, or visual disturbances. So use caution when performing tasks that require concentration.

Possible Side Effects

Nausea; headache; loss of appetite; vomiting; stomach pain; gas; impotence; changes in bowel movements; rash; thirst; dry mouth; dizziness; coughing.

Possible Adverse Effects

Notify your doctor if you experience muscular weakness, fatigue, or muscle cramps.

Drug Interactions

Lithium should not be taken with amiloride hydrochloride, since the combination may result in lithium toxicity.

Avoid using other potassium-sparing drugs (i.e., spironolactone or triamterene) or potassium supplements.

Usual Dose

Initial dose: 5 mg. daily.
Maintenance dose: 5 mg. to 10 mg. daily.

Overdosage

No data available.

Generic Name
Atenolol

Brand Name

Tenormin

Type of Drug

Beta blocker

Prescribed for

The treatment of hypertension as the first step or when diuretics have failed to lower blood pressure. Frequently, beta blockers are prescribed in combination with other antihypertensive medications.

Cautions and Warnings

Notify your doctor if you experience sore throat; fever; difficulty in breathing; night cough; swelling of the arms or legs; slow pulse rate; dizziness; light-headedness; confusion; depression; skin rash; unusual bleeding or bruising.

Atenolol should be used with care if you have a history of asthma or upper respiratory disease, seasonal allergies, or other respiratory conditions. These conditions may be worsened by atenolol. Atenolol may also aggravate congestive heart failure.

Do not take atenolol if you are allergic to any other beta blocker.

Diabetics should use atenolol with caution because it may mask signs of hypoglycemia or alter blood glucose levels.

Do NOT suddenly stop taking atenolol. Sudden cessation may result in angina (chest pain) or a worsening of any thyroid problems. Withdrawal from atenolol should be gradual and under a doctor's direction.

Atenolol may mask signs of hyperthyroidism and give the false impression that a thyroid condition is improving.

Use atenolol with caution if you suffer from kidney or liver disease.

Safety for use during pregnancy has not been established. Pregnant women should use atenolol only if the potential benefits clearly outweigh the unknown potential hazards to the fetus.

Mothers should not breast-feed while taking atenolol.

Atenolol may make you tired, so use caution

when driving or performing tasks that require concentration.

Possible Side Effects

Light-headedness; insomnia; weakness; fatigue; visual disturbances; hallucinations; disorientation; short-term memory loss; nausea; vomiting; stomach upset; abdominal cramping and diarrhea; constipation.

Possible Adverse Effects

Decreased heart rate; excessively low blood pressure; tingling in the extremities; fainting; difficulty in breathing; chest pain.

Drug Interactions

Do not take atenolol in combination with MAO inhibitors (there should be a 2-week period between the cessation of MAO inhibitor therapy and the start of beta-blocker treatment).

Atenolol may increase the effectiveness of insulin or oral antidiabetic drugs. If you are diabetic, discuss the situation with your doctor, who will probably reduce the dosage of your antidiabetic medication.

Atenolol may alter the effectiveness of digitalis on your heart. The digitalis dosage may have to be changed.

Atenolol may increase the effects of other antihypertensive medications. Usually this interaction has positive results, but it may require your doctor to adjust the dosage of your other antihypertensive medications.

While taking atenolol, do not use over-the-counter cough, cold, or allergy medications unless these products have been approved by your doctor or pharmacist.

The effects of atenolol may be reversed by isoproterenol, norepinephrine, dopamine, or dobutamine.

Usual Dose

Initial dose: 50 mg. once daily.
Maintenance dose: 50 to 100 mg. once daily.
(Patients with kidney disease may need only 50 mg. every other day.)

Overdosage

Symptoms are slowed heart rate, heart failure, excessively low blood pressure, and spasms of the bronchial muscles, which make it difficult to breathe. If you think you are experiencing an overdose, contact your doctor immediately, or go to a hospital emergency room. ALWAYS bring the medicine bottle with you.

Generic Name
Bendroflumethiazide

Brand Name

Naturetin

Type of Drug

Thiazide diuretic

Prescribed for

The initial treatment of hypertension. May be administered with other antihypertensive medications.

Cautions and Warnings

Do not take bendroflumethiazide if you are allergic or sensitive to it, to other diuretics, or to sulfa drugs. This diuretic contains tartrazine, a substance that can cause allergic reactions, especially if you are allergic to aspirin.

Although diuretics have been used to treat specific conditions in pregnancy, in general use by pregnant women should be avoided. Bendroflumethiazide can cross the placental barrier and pass into the unborn child, creating the potential for problems. Diuretics are also found in the breast milk of nursing mothers.

Use bendroflumethiazide with caution if you suffer from kidney or liver disease.

Bendroflumethiazide may activate or worsen gout or lupus (systemic lupus erythematosus).

Bendroflumethiazide will increase urination, so you should take it early in the day.

To avoid upset stomach, take the pills with food or milk.

Possible Side Effects

Bendroflumethiazide may cause an electrolyte imbalance (potassium loss) in the body. *Signs of low potassium levels* are: dryness of the mouth; thirst; weakness; lethargy; drowsiness; restlessness; muscle pains or cramps; gout; muscle fatigue; decreased frequency of urination and amount of urine; abnormal heart rate; stomach upset (including nausea and vomiting).

To treat this, potassium supplements are available in the form of tablets, liquids, or powders; or your doctor may suggest increased consumption of potassium-rich foods such as bananas, citrus fruits, melons, and tomatoes.

Possible Adverse Effects

Loss of appetite; stomach upset; nausea; vomiting; cramping; diarrhea; constipation; dizziness; headache; tingling of the toes and fingers; restlessness; changes in blood composition; sensitivity to sunlight; rash; itching; fever; difficulty in breathing; allergic reactions; dizziness when rising quickly from a sitting or lying position; muscle spasms; weakness; blurred vision. Rare incidents of impotence have also been reported.

Drug Interactions

Bendroflumethiazide may make the action of other blood-pressure-lowering drugs more effective. This is almost always a beneficial action, but your doctor may want to lower your dosage of the other antihypertensive drug.

The possibility of developing imbalances in body fluids and electrolytes is increased if you take certain medications—such as digitalis or adrenal corticosteroids—while you take bendroflumethiazide.

If you are taking an oral antidiabetic drug and begin taking bendroflumethiazide, the antidiabetic dose may have to be adjusted. Insulin requirements may also be affected.

Lithium carbonate should not be taken with diuretics because the combination may increase the risk of lithium toxicity.

If you are taking bendroflumethiazide, avoid over-the-counter medications for the treatment of coughs, colds, and allergies, which may contain stimulants that raise your blood pressure. If you are unsure about which contain stimulants, ask your doctor or pharmacist.

Usual Dose

Initial dose: 5 to 20 mg. daily.
Maintenance dose: 2.5 to 15 mg. daily.

Overdosage

Symptoms are fatigue, confusion, dizziness, nausea, lethargy, and coma. If you think you are experiencing an overdose, contact your doctor immediately, or go to a hospital emergency room. ALWAYS bring the medicine bottle with you.

Generic Name
Benzthiazide

Brand Names

Aquatag
Exna
Hydrex
Marazide
Proaqua
(Also available in generic form)

Type of Drug

Thiazide diuretic

Prescribed for

The initial treatment of hypertension. May be administered with other antihypertensive medications.

Cautions and Warnings

Do not take benzthiazide if you are allergic or sensitive to it, to other diuretics, or to sulfa drugs.

Some diuretics contain tartrazine, a substance that can cause allergic reactions, especially if you are allergic to aspirin.

Although diuretics have been used to treat specific conditions in pregnancy, in general use by pregnant women should be avoided. Benzthiazide can cross the placental barrier and pass into the unborn child, creating the potential for problems. Diuretics are also found in the breast milk of nursing mothers.

Use benzthiazide with caution if you suffer from kidney or liver disease.

Benzthiazide may activate or worsen gout or lupus (systemic lupus erythematosus).

Benzthiazide will increase urination, so you should take it early in the day.

To avoid upset stomach, take the pills with food or milk.

Possible Side Effects

Benzthiazide may cause an electrolyte imbalance (potassium loss) in the body. *Signs of low potassium levels* are: dryness of the mouth; thirst; weakness; lethargy; drowsiness; restlessness; muscle pains or cramps; gout; muscle fatigue; decreased frequency of urination and amount of urine; abnormal heart rate; stomach upset (including nausea and vomiting).

To treat this, potassium supplements are available in the form of tablets, liquids, or powders; or your doctor may suggest increased consumption of potassium-rich foods such as bananas, citrus fruits, melons, and tomatoes.

Possible Adverse Effects

Loss of appetite; stomach upset; nausea; vomiting; cramping; diarrhea; constipation; dizziness;

headache; tingling of the toes and fingers; restlessness; changes in blood composition; sensitivity to sunlight; rash; itching; fever; difficulty in breathing; allergic reactions; dizziness when rising quickly from a sitting or lying position; muscle spasms; weakness; blurred vision. Rare incidents of impotence have also been reported.

Drug Interactions

Benzthiazide may make the action of other blood-pressure-lowering drugs more effective. This is almost always a beneficial action, but your doctor may want to lower your dosage of the other antihypertensive drug.

The possibility of developing imbalances in body fluids and electrolytes is increased if you take certain medications—such as digitalis or adrenal corticosteroids—while you take benzthiazide.

If you are taking an oral antidiabetic drug and begin taking benzthiazide, the antidiabetic dose may have to be adjusted. Insulin requirements may also be affected.

Lithium carbonate should not be taken with diuretics because the combination may increase the risk of lithium toxicity.

If you are taking benzthiazide, avoid over-the-counter medications for the treatment of coughs, colds, and allergies, which may contain stimulants that raise your blood pressure. If you are unsure about which contain stimulants, ask your doctor or pharmacist.

Usual Dose

Initial dose: 50 to 100 mg. daily.
Maintenance dose: may range up to 200 mg.

Overdosage

Symptoms are fatigue, confusion, dizziness, nausea, lethargy, and coma. If you think you are experiencing an overdose, contact your doctor immediately, or go to a hospital emergency room. ALWAYS bring the medicine bottle with you.

Generic Name
Bumetanide

Brand Name

Bumex

Type of Drug

Loop diuretic

Prescribed for

The treatment of hypertension. May be administered with other antihypertensive medications.

Cautions and Warnings

Do not take bumetanide if you are allergic or sensitive to it, to other diuretics, or to sulfa drugs.

Although diuretics have been used to treat specific conditions in pregnancy, in general use by pregnant women should be avoided. Bumetanide can cross the placental barrier and pass into the unborn child, creating the potential for problems. Diuretics are also found in the breast milk of nursing mothers.

Use bumetanide with caution if you suffer from kidney or liver disease.

Bumetanide may activate or worsen gout or lupus (systemic lupus erythematosus).

Bumetanide will increase urination, so you should take it early in the day.

To avoid upset stomach, take the pills with food or milk.

Possible Side Effects

Bumetanide may cause an electrolyte imbalance (potassium loss) in the body. *Signs of low potassium levels* are: dryness of the mouth; thirst; weakness; lethargy; drowsiness; restlessness; muscle pains or cramps; gout; muscle fatigue; decreased frequency of urination and amount of urine; abnormal heart rate; stomach upset (including nausea and vomiting).

To treat this, potassium supplements are available in the form of tablets, liquids, or powders; or your doctor may suggest increased consumption of potassium-rich foods such as bananas, citrus fruits, melons, and tomatoes.

Possible Adverse Effects

Loss of appetite; stomach upset; nausea; vomiting; cramping; diarrhea; constipation; dizziness; headache; tingling of the toes and fingers; restlessness; changes in blood composition; sensitivity to sunlight; rash; itching; fever; difficulty in breathing; allergic reactions; dizziness when rising quickly from a sitting or lying position; muscle spasms; weakness; blurred vision. Rare incidents of impotence have also been reported.

Drug Interactions

Bumetanide may make the action of other blood-pressure-lowering drugs more effective. This is almost always a beneficial action, but your doctor may want to lower your dosage of the other antihypertensive drug.

The possibility of developing imbalances in body fluids and electrolytes is increased if you take certain medications—such as digitalis or adrenal corticosteroids—while you take bumetanide.

If you are taking an oral antidiabetic drug and begin taking bumetanide, the antidiabetic dose may have to be adjusted. Insulin requirements may also be affected.

Lithium carbonate should not be taken with diuretics because the combination may increase the risk of lithium toxicity.

If you are taking bumetanide, avoid over-the-counter medications for the treatment of coughs, colds, and allergies, which may contain stimulants that raise your blood pressure. If you are unsure about which contain stimulants, ask your doctor or pharmacist.

Usual Dose

Initial dose: 0.5 to 2 mg. daily.
Maintenance dose: 0.5 to 10 mg.

Overdosage

Symptoms are fatigue, dehydration, profound water loss, confusion, dizziness, lethargy, and coma. If you think you are experiencing an overdose, contact your doctor immediately, or go to a hospital emergency room. ALWAYS bring the medicine bottle with you.

Generic Name
Captopril

Brand Name

Capoten

Type of Drug

ACE Inhibitor

Prescribed for

The treatment of hypertension that has not responded to other antihypertensive medications.

Cautions and Warnings

Take 1 hour before meals.

Captopril can cause kidney disease, especially notable by loss of protein in the urine. Patients should have the amount of protein in their urine measured monthly for the first 9 months and every few months afterward.

Captopril can also cause reduction in the white-blood-cell count. This can result in increased susceptibility to infection.

Captopril should be used with caution by people who have kidney disease, diseases of the immune/collagen system (particularly lupus), or who have taken other drugs that affect the white-blood-cell count.

Captopril should be used by children, pregnant women, or breast-feeding mothers *only* when absolutely necessary.

Do NOT stop taking captopril unless directed to do so by your doctor.

Notify your doctor if you experience mouth sores; sore throat; swelling of the hands or feet; fever;

irregular heartbeat; chest pains; persistent skin rash; impaired taste perception; vomiting; excessive perspiration; dehydration; diarrhea.

Avoid sudden changes in posture to lessen the chances of becoming dizzy.

Avoid cough, cold, or allergy medications unless they have been approved by your doctor or pharmacist.

Possible Side Effects

Rash (usually mild); itching; fever; loss of taste perception (usually returns in 2 to 3 months).

Possible Adverse Effects

Adverse effects on the kidney, causing loss of protein in the urine, kidney failure, excessive or frequent urination, and reduction in the amount of urine produced; adverse effects on the blood system, especially white blood cells; swelling of the face, of the mucous membranes of the mouth, or of the arms and legs; flushing or pale skin; excessively low blood pressure; chest pain; abnormal heartbeat; spasm of the blood vessels; heart failure.

Drug Interactions

The effect of captopril on blood pressure is increased with diuretics. While this is normally beneficial to you, it is important that you follow your doctor's advice closely, especially when taking the first combined dose of a diuretic and captopril.

Use vasodilators, spironolactone, triamterene, amiloride hydrochloride, or potassium supplements with caution in combination with captopril.

Usual Dose

Initial dose: 25 mg. 3 times daily.
Maintenance dose: 25 to 150 mg. 3 times daily.

Overdosage

No data available.

Generic Name
Chlorothiazide

Brand Names

Diachlor
Diuril
(Also available in generic form)

Type of Drug

Thiazide diuretic

Prescribed for

The initial treatment of hypertension. May be administered with other antihypertensive medications.

Cautions and Warnings

Do not take chlorothiazide if you are allergic or sensitive to it, to other diuretics, or to sulfa drugs.

Although diuretics have been used to treat specific conditions in pregnancy, in general use by pregnant women should be avoided. Chlorothiazide can cross the placental barrier and pass into the unborn child, creating the potential for problems. Diuretics are also found in the breast milk of nursing mothers.

Use chlorothiazide with caution if you suffer from kidney or liver disease.

Chlorothiazide may activate or worsen gout or lupus (systemic lupus erythematosus).

Chlorothiazide will increase urination, so you should take it early in the day.

To avoid upset stomach, take the pills with food or milk.

Possible Side Effects

Chlorothiazide may cause an electrolyte imbalance (potassium loss) in the body. *Signs of low potassium levels* are: dryness of the mouth; thirst; weakness; lethargy; drowsiness; restlessness; muscle pains or cramps; gout; muscle fatigue; decreased frequency of urination and amount of urine; abnormal heart rate; stomach upset (including nausea and vomiting).

To treat this, potassium supplements are available in the form of tablets, liquids, or powders; or your doctor may suggest increased consumption of potassium-rich foods such as bananas, citrus fruits, melons, and tomatoes.

Possible Adverse Effects

Loss of appetite; stomach upset; nausea; vomiting; cramping; diarrhea; constipation; dizziness; headache; tingling of the toes and fingers; restlessness; changes in blood composition; sensitivity to sunlight; rash; itching; fever; difficulty in breathing; allergic reactions; dizziness when rising quickly from a sitting or lying position; muscle spasms; weakness; blurred vision. Rare incidents of impotence have also been reported.

Drug Interactions

Chlorothiazide may make the action of other

blood-pressure-lowering drugs more effective. This is almost always a beneficial action, but your doctor may want to lower your dosage of the other antihypertensive drug.

The possibility of developing imbalances in body fluids and electrolytes is increased if you take certain medications—such as digitalis or adrenal cortico-steroids—while you take chlorothiazide.

If you are taking an oral antidiabetic drug and begin taking chlorothiazide, the antidiabetic dose may have to be adjusted. Insulin requirements may also be affected.

Lithium carbonate should not be taken with diuretics because the combination may increase the risk of lithium toxicity.

If you are taking chlorothiazide, avoid over-the-counter medications for the treatment of coughs, colds, and allergies, which may contain stimulants that raise your blood pressure. If you are unsure about which contain stimulants, ask your doctor or pharmacist.

Usual Dose

Initial dose: 0.5 to 2 grams daily.

Maintenance dose: may be increased or decreased according to your response to the medication.

Overdosage

Symptoms are fatigue, confusion, dizziness, nausea, lethargy, and coma. If you think you are experiencing an overdose, contact your doctor immediately, or go to a hospital emergency room. ALWAYS bring the medicine bottle with you.

Generic Name
Chlorthalidone

Brand Names

Hygroton
Hylidone
Thalitone
(Also available in generic form)

Type of Drug

Thiazidelike diuretic

Prescribed for

The initial treatment of hypertension. May be administered with other antihypertensive medications.

Cautions and Warnings

Do not take chlorthalidone if you are allergic or sensitive to it, or to other diuretics, or to sulfa drugs.

Although diuretics have been used to treat specific conditions in pregnancy, in general use by pregnant women should be avoided. Chlorthalidone can cross the placental barrier and pass into the unborn child, creating the potential for problems. Diuretics are also found in the breast milk of nursing mothers.

Use chlorthalidone with caution if you suffer from kidney or liver disease.

Chlorthalidone may activate or worsen gout or lupus (systemic lupus erythematosus).

Chlorthalidone will increase urination, so you should take it early in the day.

To avoid upset stomach, take the pills with food or milk.

Possible Side Effects

Chlorthalidone may cause an electrolyte imbalance (potassium loss) in the body. *Signs of low potassium levels* are: dryness of the mouth; thirst; weakness; lethargy; drowsiness; restlessness; muscle pains or cramps; gout; muscle fatigue; decreased frequency of urination and amount of urine; abnormal heart rate; stomach upset (including nausea and vomiting).

To treat this, potassium supplements are available in the form of tablets, liquids, or powders; or your doctor may suggest increased consumption of potassium-rich foods such as bananas, citrus fruits, melons, and tomatoes.

Possible Adverse Effects

Loss of appetite; stomach upset; nausea; vomiting; cramping; diarrhea; constipation; dizziness; headache; tingling of the toes and fingers; restlessness; changes in blood composition; sensitivity to sunlight; rash; itching; fever; difficulty in breathing; allergic reactions; dizziness when rising quickly from a sitting or lying position; muscle spasms; weakness; blurred vision. Rare incidents of impotence have also been reported.

Drug Interactions

Chlorthalidone may make the action of other blood-pressure-lowering drugs more effective. This is almost always a beneficial action, but your doctor may want to lower your dosage of the other antihypertensive drug.

The possibility of developing imbalances in body fluids and electrolytes is increased if you take certain medications—such as digitalis or adrenal corticosteroids—while you take chlorthalidone.

If you are taking an oral antidiabetic drug and begin taking chlorthalidone, the antidiabetic dose may have to be adjusted. Insulin requirements may also be affected.

Lithium carbonate should not be taken with diuretics because the combination may increase the risk of lithium toxicity.

If you are taking chlorthalidone, avoid over-the-counter medications for the treatment of coughs, colds, and allergies, which may contain stimulants that raise your blood pressure. If you are unsure about which products contain stimulants, ask your doctor or pharmacist.

Usual Dose

Initial dose: 25 mg. once daily.
Maintenance dose: adjusted to suit your needs.

Overdosage

Symptoms are fatigue, confusion, dizziness, nausea, lethargy, and coma. If you think you are experiencing an overdose, contact your doctor immediately, or go to a hospital emergency room. ALWAYS bring the medicine bottle with you.

Generic Name
Clonidine Hydrochloride

Brand Name

Catapres

Type of Drug

Antiadrenergic agent

Prescribed for

The treatment of hypertension—either alone or with other antihypertensive medications.

Cautions and Warnings

Abruptly stopping your clonidine hydrochloride therapy may result in a sudden rise in your blood pressure. Rare instances of death have been reported upon sudden cessation of clonidine hydrochloride therapy. Do NOT stop taking your clonidine hydrochloride unless told to do so by your doctor. Usually your doctor will gradually reduce your dosage over a period of 2–4 days.

Some people develop a tolerance to the usual doses of clonidine hydrochloride. If this happens to you, your blood pressure may increase, and you will require a change in dosage.

Clonidine hydrochloride is not recommended for use by pregnant women or those who intend to become pregnant. Nursing mothers should not breast-feed while taking this drug.

Clonidine hydrochloride may cause drowsiness. Be extremely careful while driving or performing tasks that require concentration.

Avoid taking cough, cold, or allergy medications unless directed to do so by your doctor.

Possible Side Effects

Dry mouth; drowsiness; sedation; constipation; dizziness; headache; fatigue. These effects tend to diminish as you continue taking clonidine hydrochloride.

Possible Adverse Effects

Nausea; loss of appetite; feeling of illness; vomiting; weight gain; breast enlargement; various effects on the heart; changes in dream patterns; nightmares; difficulty in sleeping; nervousness; restlessness; anxiety; mental depression; rash; hives; itching; thinning or loss of scalp hair; difficulty in urinating; impotence; dryness or burning of the eyes.

Drug Interactions

Clonidine hydrochloride has a depressive effect and will increase the depressive effects of alcohol, barbiturates, sedatives, and tranquilizers. Avoid them when taking clonidine hydrochloride.

Tolazoline and tricyclic antidepressants may inhibit the effectiveness of clonidine hydrochloride.

Usual Dose

Initial dose: 0.1 mg. twice daily.
Maintenance dose: 0.2 to 0.8 mg. in divided daily doses.

Overdosage

Symptoms include severe lowering of blood pressure (i.e., fainting, extreme dizziness), weakness, and vomiting. If you think you are experiencing an overdose, contact your doctor immediately, or go to a hospital emergency room. ALWAYS bring the medicine bottle with you.

Generic Name
Cyclothiazide

Brand Names

Anhydron
Fluidil

Type of Drug

Thiazide diuretic

Prescribed for

The initial treatment of hypertension. May be administered with other antihypertensive medications.

Cautions and Warnings

Do not take cyclothiazide if you are allergic or sensitive to it, to other diuretics, or to sulfa drugs.

Although diuretics have been used to treat specific conditions in pregnancy, in general use by pregnant women should be avoided. Cyclothiazide can cross the placental barrier and pass into the unborn child, creating the potential for problems. Diuretics are also found in the breast milk of nursing mothers.

Use cyclothiazide with caution if you suffer from kidney or liver disease.

Cyclothiazide may activate or worsen gout or lupus (systemic lupus erythematosus).

Cyclothiazide will increase urination, so you should take it early in the day.

To avoid upset stomach, take the pills with food or milk.

Possible Side Effects

Cyclothiazide may cause an electrolyte imbalance (potassium loss) in the body. *Signs of low potassium levels* are: dryness of the mouth; thirst; weakness; lethargy; drowsiness; restlessness; muscle pains or cramps; gout; muscle fatigue; decreased frequency of urination and amount of urine; abnormal heart rate; stomach upset (including nausea and vomiting).

To treat this, potassium supplements are available in the form of tablets, liquids, or powders; or your doctor may suggest increased consumption of potassium-rich foods such as bananas, citrus fruits, melons, and tomatoes.

Possible Adverse Effects

Loss of appetite; stomach upset; nausea; vomiting; cramping; diarrhea; constipation; dizziness; headache; tingling of the toes and fingers; restlessness; changes in blood composition; sensitivity to sunlight; rash; itching; fever; difficulty in breathing; allergic reactions; dizziness when rising quickly from a sitting or lying position; muscle spasms; weakness; blurred vision. Rare incidents of impotence have also been reported.

Drug Interactions

Cyclothiazide may make the action of other blood-pressure-lowering drugs more effective. This is almost always a beneficial action, but your doctor may want to lower your dosage of the other antihypertensive drug.

The possibility of developing imbalances in body fluids and electrolytes is increased if you take certain medications—such as digitalis or adrenal corticosteroids—while you take cyclothiazide.

If you are taking an oral antidiabetic drug and begin taking cyclothiazide, the antidiabetic dose may have to be adjusted. Insulin requirements may also be affected.

Lithium carbonate should not be taken with diuretics because the combination may increase the risk of lithium toxicity.

If you are taking cyclothiazide, avoid over-the-counter medications for the treatment of coughs, colds, and allergies, which may contain stimulants that raise your blood pressure. If you are unsure about which contain stimulants, ask your doctor or pharmacist.

Usual Dose

Initial dose: 2 mg. daily.
Maintenance dose: may be adjusted to 4 to 6 mg. daily.

Overdosage

Symptoms are fatigue, confusion, dizziness, nausea, lethargy, and coma. If you think you are experiencing an overdose, contact your doctor immediately, or go to a hospital emergency room. ALWAYS bring the medicine bottle with you.

Generic Name
Deserpidine

Brand Name

Harmonyl

Type of Drug

Antiadrenergic agent

Prescribed for

The treatment of hypertension—either alone or with other antihypertensive medications.

Cautions and Warnings

Do not stop taking deserpidine unless directed to do so by your doctor.

Use with extreme caution if you suffer from depression, since deserpidine may induce severe depression that may persist for several months after you stop taking it. Notify your doctor if you experience any changes in mood or sleep habits, or continual severe stomach pain.

Avoid cough, cold, or allergy medications except when they are approved by your doctor or pharmacist.

If dizziness occurs, avoid suddenly rising from a sitting or reclining position.

Pregnant women should use deserpidine only when the potential benefits clearly outweigh the unknown potential hazards to the fetus.

Mothers should not breast-feed when taking deserpidine.

Use deserpidine with caution if you suffer from kidney or liver disease or have a history of peptic ulcers, ulcerative colitis, or gallstones.

This product contains tartrazine, a substance found to cause allergic reactions, especially in people allergic to aspirin.

Possible Side Effects

Stuffy nose; dry mouth; dizziness; headache; breathing difficulties; impotence or decreased sex drive; muscle aches; weight gain; breast enlargement; lactation (in females).

Possible Adverse Effects

Nausea; vomiting; loss of appetite; diarrhea; stomach bleeding; chest pain; abnormal heart rhythms; swelling of hands or feet; depression; fainting; involuntary movements or twitching of the head and neck.

Drug Interactions

Digitalis and quinidine, when used with deserpidine, may cause abnormal heart rhythms.

MAO inhibitors should be avoided or used with extreme caution.

Deserpidine, when used with beta blockers, may result in extreme low blood pressure manifested by fainting, vertigo, or dizziness when suddenly rising from a sitting or reclining position.

Usual Dose

Initial dose: 0.75 to 1 mg. daily.
Maintenance dose: 0.25 mg. once daily.

Overdosage

Symptoms are changes in consciousness ranging from dizziness to coma; diarrhea; difficulty in breathing; slow heartbeat; flushing of the skin; pupil constriction. If you think you are experiencing an overdose, call your doctor immediately, or go to a hospital emergency room. ALWAYS bring the medicine bottle with you.

Brand Name
Dyazide

Ingredients

Hydrochlorothiazide
Triamterene

Type of Drug

Antihypertensive medication combining a thiazide diuretic (hydrochlorothiazide) with a potassium-sparing diuretic (triamterene).

Prescribed for

The treatment of hypertension when it is necessary to counteract the potassium loss caused by diuretics.

Cautions and Warnings

Do not take Dyazide if you have severe kidney disease, if you may be allergic to this drug or to any sulfa drug, or if you have a history of allergy or bronchial asthma. Dyazide may be used to treat specific conditions in pregnant women, but the decision to use this medication by pregnant women should be weighed carefully because the drug may cross the placental barrier and pass into the blood of the unborn child. Dyazide may appear in the breast milk of nursing mothers. Do not take any potassium supplements together with Dyazide unless specifically directed to do so by your doctor.

Take Dyazide exactly as prescribed.

Possible Side Effects

Drowsiness; lethargy; headache; upset stomach; cramping and diarrhea; rash; mental confusion; fever; feeling of ill health; enlargement of the breasts; inability to achieve or maintain erection (in males); irregular menstrual cycles or deepening of the voice (in females).

Possible Adverse Effects

Loss of appetite; headache; tingling in the toes and fingers; restlessness; anemias or other effects on components of the blood; unusual sensitivity to sunlight; dizziness when rising quickly from a sitting position. Dyazide can also produce muscle spasms, gout, weakness, and blurred vision.

Drug Interactions

Dyazide may make the action of other blood-pressure-lowering drugs more effective. This is almost always a beneficial action, but your doctor may want to lower your dosage of the other antihypertensive drug.

The possibility of developing imbalances in body fluids and electrolytes is increased if you take other medications—such as digitalis and adrenal corticosteroids—while you are taking Dyazide.

If you are taking an oral antidiabetic drug and begin taking Dyazide, the antidiabetic dose may have to be altered.

Lithium carbonate should not be taken with Dyazide because the combination may increase the risk of lithium toxicity.

Avoid over-the-counter cough, cold, or allergy remedies containing stimulant drugs that can aggravate your condition.

Usual Dose

1 to 2 tablets twice daily.

Overdosage

Symptoms are fatigue, dizziness, nausea, vomiting, weakness, lethargy, and coma. If you think you are experiencing an overdose, contact your doctor immediately, or go to a hospital emergency room. ALWAYS bring the medicine bottle with you.

Generic Name
Ethacrynic Acid

Brand Name

Edecrin

Type of Drug

Loop diuretic

Prescribed for

The treatment of hypertension. May be administered with other antihypertensive medications.

Cautions and Warnings

Do not take ethacrynic acid if you are allergic or
sensitive to it, to other diuretics, or to sulfa drugs.

Although diuretics have been used to treat specific conditions in pregnancy, in general use by
pregnant women should be avoided. Ethacrynic
acid can cross the placental barrier and pass into
the unborn child, creating the potential for problems.
Diuretics are also found in the breast milk of nursing mothers.

Use ethacrynic acid with caution if you suffer
from kidney or liver disease.

Ethacrynic acid may activate or worsen gout or
lupus (systemic lupus erythematosus).

Ethacrynic acid will increase urination, so you
should take it early in the day.

To avoid upset stomach, take the pills with food
or milk.

Possible Side Effects

Ethacrynic acid may cause an electrolyte imbalance (potassium loss) in the body. *Signs of low potassium levels* are: dryness of the mouth; thirst; weakness; lethargy; drowsiness; restlessness; muscle pains or cramps; gout; muscle fatigue; decreased frequency of urination and amount of urine; abnormal heart rate; stomach upset (including nausea and vomiting).

To treat this, potassium supplements are available in the form of tablets, liquids, or powders; or your doctor may suggest increased consumption of potassium-rich foods such as bananas, citrus fruits, melons, and tomatoes.

Possible Adverse Effects

Loss of appetite; stomach upset; nausea; vomiting; cramping; diarrhea; constipation; dizziness; headache; tingling of the toes and fingers; restlessness; changes in blood composition; sensitivity to sunlight; rash; itching; fever; difficulty in breathing; allergic reactions; dizziness when rising quickly from a sitting or lying position; muscle spasms; weakness; blurred vision. Rare incidents of impotence have also been reported.

Drug Interactions

Ethacrynic acid may make the action of other blood-pressure-lowering drugs more effective. This is almost always a beneficial action, but your doctor may want to lower your dosage of the other antihypertensive drug.

The possibility of developing imbalances in body fluids and electrolytes is increased if you take certain medications—such as digitalis or adrenal corticosteroids—while you take ethacrynic acid.

If you are taking an oral antidiabetic drug and begin taking ethacrynic acid, the antidiabetic dose may have to be adjusted. Insulin requirements may also be affected.

Lithium carbonate should not be taken with diuretics because the combination may increase the risk of lithium toxicity.

If you are taking ethacrynic acid, avoid over-the-counter medications for the treatment of coughs, colds, and allergies, which may contain stimulants that raise your blood pressure. If you are unsure about which contain stimulants, ask your doctor or pharmacist.

Usual Dose

Initial dose: 50 to 100 mg. daily.
Maintenance dose: adjusted to suit your needs.

Overdosage

Symptoms are fatigue, dehydration, profound water loss, dizziness, confusion, lethargy, and coma. If you think you are experiencing an overdose, contact your doctor immediately, or go to a hospital emergency room. ALWAYS bring the medicine bottle with you.

Generic Name
Furosemide

Brand Name

Lasix
(Also available in generic form)

Type of Drug

Loop diuretic

Prescribed for

The treatment of hypertension. May be administered with other antihypertensive medications.

Cautions and Warnings

Do not take furosemide if you are allergic or sensitive to it, to other diuretics, or to sulfa drugs.

Although diuretics have been used to treat specific conditions in pregnancy, in general use by pregnant women should be avoided. Furosemide can cross the placental barrier and pass into the unborn child, creating the potential for problems. Diuretics are also found in the breast milk of nursing mothers.

Use furosemide with caution if you suffer from kidney or liver disease.

Furosemide may activate or worsen gout or lupus (systemic lupus erythematosus).

Furosemide will increase urination, so you should take it early in the day.

To avoid upset stomach, take the pills with food or milk.

Do not expose furosemide tablets to light, as light will discolor them. Do NOT use discolored tablets.

Possible Side Effects

Furosemide may cause an electrolyte imbalance (potassium loss) in the body. *Signs of low potassium levels* are: dryness of the mouth; thirst; weakness; lethargy; drowsiness; restlessness; muscle pains or cramps; gout; muscle fatigue; decreased frequency of urination and amount of urine; abnormal heart rate; stomach upset (including nausea and vomiting).

To treat this, potassium supplements are avail-

HIGH BLOOD PRESSURE

Drugs In Alphabetical Order

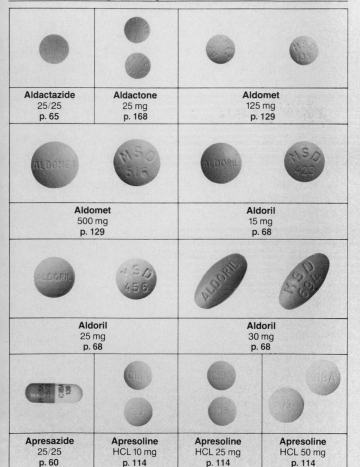

Aldactazide 25/25 p. 65	**Aldactone** 25 mg p. 168	**Aldomet** 125 mg p. 129	
Aldomet 500 mg p. 129		**Aldoril** 15 mg p. 68	
Aldoril 25 mg p. 68		**Aldoril** 30 mg p. 68	
Apresazide 25/25 p. 60	**Apresoline** HCL 10 mg p. 114	**Apresoline** HCL 25 mg p. 114	**Apresoline** HCL 50 mg p. 114

A

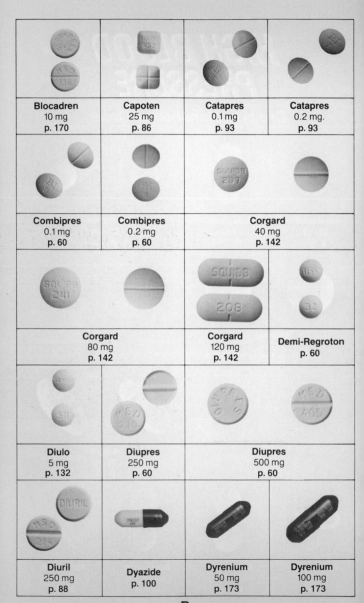

Blocadren 10 mg p. 170	**Capoten** 25 mg p. 86	**Catapres** 0.1 mg p. 93	**Catapres** 0.2 mg. p. 93
Combipres 0.1 mg p. 60	**Combipres** 0.2 mg p. 60	**Corgard** 40 mg p. 142	
Corgard 80 mg p. 142		**Corgard** 120 mg p. 142	**Demi-Regroton** p. 60
Diulo 5 mg p. 132	**Diupres** 250 mg p. 60	**Diupres** 500 mg p. 60	
Diuril 250 mg p. 88	**Dyazide** p. 100	**Dyrenium** 50 mg p. 173	**Dyrenium** 100 mg p. 173

B

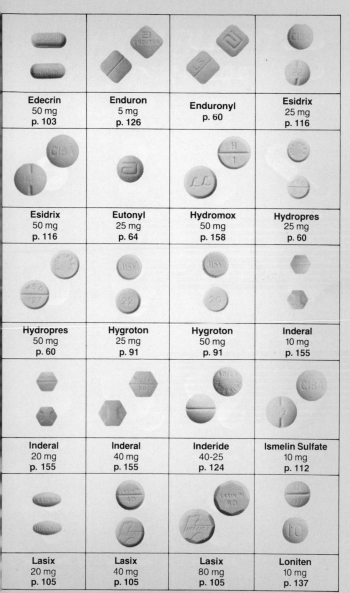

Edecrin 50 mg p. 103	**Enduron** 5 mg p. 126	**Enduronyl** p. 60	**Esidrix** 25 mg p. 116
Esidrix 50 mg p. 116	**Eutonyl** 25 mg p. 64	**Hydromox** 50 mg p. 158	**Hydropres** 25 mg p. 60
Hydropres 50 mg p. 60	**Hygroton** 25 mg p. 91	**Hygroton** 50 mg p. 91	**Inderal** 10 mg p. 155
Inderal 20 mg p. 155	**Inderal** 40 mg p. 155	**Inderide** 40-25 p. 124	**Ismelin Sulfate** 10 mg p. 112
Lasix 20 mg p. 105	**Lasix** 40 mg p. 105	**Lasix** 80 mg p. 105	**Loniten** 10 mg p. 137

C

Lopressor 50 mg p. 134	**Lopressor** 100 mg p. 134	**Minipress** 1 mg p. 153	**Minipress** 2 mg p. 153
Minipress 5 mg p. 153	**Moduretic** p. 139	**Naturetin** 5 mg p. 77	**Raudixin** 100 mg p. 178
Rauwiloid p. 70	**Regroton** p. 60	**Renese** 1 mg p. 148	**Renese** 4 mg p. 148
Salutensin p. 60	**Serpasil - Apresoline** p. 60	**Ser-Ap-Es** p. 166	**Tenormin** 50 mg p. 74
Tenormin 100 mg p. 74	**Zaroxolyn** 2.5 mg p. 132	**Zaroxolyn** 5 mg p. 132	**Zaroxolyn** 10 mg p. 132

D

able in the form of tablets, liquids, or powders; or your doctor may suggest increased consumption of potassium-rich foods such as bananas, citrus fruits, melons, and tomatoes.

Possible Adverse Effects

Loss of appetite; stomach upset; nausea; vomiting; cramping; diarrhea; constipation; dizziness; headache; tingling of the toes and fingers; restlessness; changes in blood composition; sensitivity to sunlight; rash; itching; fever; difficulty in breathing; allergic reactions; dizziness when rising quickly from a sitting or lying position; muscle spasms; weakness; blurred vision. Rare incidents of impotence have also been reported. On rare occasions, furosemide has been reported to cause hearing loss.

Drug Interactions

Furosemide may make the action of other blood-pressure-lowering drugs more effective. This is almost always a beneficial action, but your doctor may want to lower your dosage of the other antihypertensive drug.

The possibility of developing imbalances in body fluids and electrolytes is increased if you take certain medications—such as digitalis or adrenal corticosteroids—while you take furosemide.

If you are taking an oral antidiabetic drug and begin taking furosemide, the antidiabetic dose may have to be adjusted. Insulin requirements may also be affected.

Lithium carbonate should not be taken with diuretics because the combination may increase the risk of lithium toxicity.

If you are taking furosemide, avoid over-the-counter medications for the treatment of coughs, colds, and allergies, which may contain stimulants that raise your blood pressure. If you are unsure about which contain stimulants, ask your doctor or pharmacist.

Usual Dose

Initial dose: 40 mg. twice daily.
Maintenance dose: adjusted to suit your needs.

Overdosage

Symptoms are fatigue, dehydration, profound water loss, dizziness, confusion, lethargy, and coma. If you think you are experiencing an overdose, contact your doctor immediately, or go to a hospital emergency room. ALWAYS bring the medicine bottle with you.

Generic Name
Guanabenz Acetate

Brand Name

Wytensin

Type of Drug

Antiadrenergic agent

Prescribed for

The treatment of hypertension—either alone or with other antihypertensive medications.

Cautions and Warnings

Guanabenz acetate may produce drowsiness—

observe caution while driving or performing tasks that require concentration. Alcohol and other depressants have a greater effect on you when you are taking guanabenz acetate.

Do not stop taking this drug unless directed to do so by your doctor.

Use guanabenz acetate with caution if you suffer from heart, kidney, or liver disease.

Pregnant women should use guanabenz acetate only when the benefits clearly outweigh the unknown potential hazards to the fetus.

Mothers should not breast-feed while taking guanabenz acetate.

Possible Side Effects

Drowsiness; dry mouth; dizziness; weakness; headache; rash.

Possible Adverse Effects

Nausea; vomiting; diarrhea; chest pain; swelling of hands and feet; abnormal heart rhythms; stuffy nose; muscle aches; blurred vision; sleep disturbances; constipation; difficulty in breathing; increased urination.

Drug Interactions

Using guanabenz acetate with alcohol or other depressants may result in increased sleepiness.

Usual Dose

Initial dose: 4 mg. twice daily.
Maintenance dose: may be increased to 32 mg. twice daily.

Overdosage

Symptoms include sleepiness, low blood pressure, lethargy, irritability, and slow heart rate. If you think you are experiencing an overdose reaction, contact your doctor immediately, or go to a hospital emergency room. ALWAYS bring the medicine bottle with you.

Generic Name

Guanadrel Sulfate

Brand Name

Hylorel

Type of Drug

Antiadrenergic agent

Prescribed for

The treatment of hypertension—either alone or with other antihypertensive medications.

Cautions and Warnings

If you are standing and feel dizzy or weak, sit or lie down immediately. Dizziness that occurs when you suddenly change position (standing or sitting up quickly) is worse in the morning, and may be worsened by alcohol, fever, hot weather, and exercise. Changes in your position should be done slowly to minimize this dizziness.

Avoid cough, cold, or allergy medications unless their use has been approved by your doctor or pharmacist.

You should not take guanadrel sulfate if you

suffer from pheochromocytoma (a form of cancerous tumor), congestive heart failure, a known sensitivity to the drug, or if you have been taking MAO inhibitors within the last week.

Use with caution if you suffer from bronchial asthma or peptic ulcers.

Possible Side Effects

Shortness of breath; palpitations; coughing; fatigue; headache; dizziness; depression; confusion; muscle aches; stomach pain; weight gain; frequent urination.

Possible Adverse Effects

Chest pain; loss of appetite; impotence; difficulty in ejaculation; sleep disturbances.

Drug Interactions

Beta blockers and reserpine may enhance the effectiveness of guanadrel sulfate.

Guanadrel sulfate increases the effects of norepinephrine.

Usual Dose

Initial dose: 10 mg. daily.
Maintenance dose: 20 to 75 mg. twice daily.

Overdosage

Symptoms are dizziness, blurred vision, and fainting (especially when standing). Other symptoms include a slow heart rate and diarrhea. If you think you are experiencing an overdose, call your doctor immediately, or go to a hospital emergency room. ALWAYS bring the medicine bottle with you.

Generic Name

Guanethidine Sulfate

Brand Name

Ismelin Sulfate

Type of Drug

Antiadrenergic agent

Prescribed for

The treatment of hypertension—either alone or with other antihypertensive medications.

Cautions and Warnings

Do not stop taking guanethidine sulfate unless directed to do so by your doctor.

Notify your doctor if you experience severe diarrhea, frequent dizziness, or fainting.

If dizziness occurs, avoid sudden changes in posture. Alcohol and heat may increase the chance of your becoming dizzy or fainting.

Patients who may be allergic to this drug, who are taking an MAO inhibitor, or who have a tumor diagnosed as pheochromocytoma should not take guanethidine sulfate.

Use guanethidine sulfate with extreme caution if you suffer from heart disease, kidney disease, a history of peptic ulcers or bronchial asthma, or encephalopathy.

This product may contain tartrazine, a substance found to cause allergic reactions, especially in people allergic to aspirin.

Pregnant women should use guanethidine sulfate only when the potential benefits clearly outweigh the unknown potential hazards to the fetus.

Possible Side Effects

Weakness (especially on rising quickly from a sitting or reclining position); slowed heartbeat; increased bowel movements; difficult ejaculation; retention of fluid in the body.

Possible Adverse Effects

Difficulty in breathing; fatigue; nausea; vomiting; increased frequency of nighttime urination; difficulty in controlling urine flow; itching; rash; loss of scalp hair; dry mouth; involuntary lowering of the eyelids; blurred vision; muscle aches and spasms; mental depression; chest pains (angina pectoris); tingling in the chest; stuffy nose; weight gain; asthma. Guanethidine sulfate may affect kidney function.

Drug Interactions

Guanethidine sulfate may interact with digitalis to slow heart rate excessively.

Guanethidine sulfate may make the action of other blood-pressure-lowering drugs more effective. This is almost always a beneficial action, but your doctor may want to lower your dosage of the other antihypertensive drug.

Drugs with stimulant properties (antidepressants, decongestants), oral contraceptives, and some antipsychotic drugs (phenothiazines, etc.) may reduce the effectiveness of guanethidine sulfate. Avoid over-the-counter cough, cold, or allergy medications unless approved by your doctor or pharmacist.

This drug should not be taken with MAO inhibitors. MAO inhibitors should be stopped at least one week before taking guanethidine sulfate.

Usual Dose

Initial dose: 10 mg. daily.
Maintenance dose: 25 to 50 mg. once daily.

Overdosage

Symptoms consist of exaggerated or prolonged side effects, including dizziness, weakness, slowed heartbeat, and diarrhea. If these symptoms appear, or if you think you are experiencing an overdose, contact your doctor immediately, or go to a hospital emergency room. ALWAYS bring the medicine bottle with you.

Generic Name
Hydralazine Hydrochloride

Brand Names

Apresoline
Dralzine
(Also available in generic form)

Type of Drug

Vasodilator

Prescribed for

The treatment of hypertension—either alone or with other antihypertensive medications.

Cautions and Warnings

Do not stop taking hydralazine hydrochloride unless directed to do so by your doctor.

Avoid cough, cold, or allergy medications unless they are approved by your doctor or pharmacist.

Some vasodilators contain tartrazine, a substance that can cause allergic reactions, especially if you are allergic to asprin.

Notify your doctor if you experience unexplained prolonged fatigue, fever, muscle or joint aching, or chest pains.

Avoid sudden changes in posture to minimize the chance of becoming dizzy.

Long-term administration of large doses of hydralazine hydrochloride may produce an arthritislike syndrome (lupus) in some people, although symptoms of this problem usually disappear when the drug is discontinued.

Use hydralazine hydrochloride with caution if you suffer from kidney disease.

Pregnant women should use hydralazine hydrochloride only when the potential benefits clearly outweigh the potential hazards to the fetus.

Mothers should not breast-feed while taking this drug.

Possible Side Effects

Headache; palpitations; loss of appetite; nausea; vomiting; diarrhea; rapid heartbeat.

Possible Adverse Effects

Stuffy nose; flushing, tearing eyes; itching and redness of the eyes; numbness and tingling of the hands and feet; dizziness; tremors; muscle cramps; depression; disorientation; anxiety; itching; rash; chills; (occasional) hepatitis; constipation; difficulty in urination; adverse effects on the blood.

Drug Interactions

Hydralazine hydrochloride should be used with caution if you are taking MAO inhibitors.

Use cough, cold, and allergy remedies with extreme caution.

Usual Dose

Initial dose: 10 mg. 4 times daily for the first 2 to 4 days. 25 mg. 4 times daily for the remainder of the first week. Second and following weeks: 50 mg. 4 times daily.
Maintenance dose: adjusted to suit your needs.

Overdosage

If symptoms of extreme low blood pressure (fainting, severe dizziness), rapid heartbeat, generalized skin flushing, chest pains, or irregular heart rhythms occur, contact your doctor immediately, or go to a hospital emergency room. ALWAYS bring the medicine bottle with you.

Generic Name
Hydrochlorothiazide

Brand Names

Aquazide H	Mictrin
Chlorzide	Oretic
Diaqua	Thiuretic
Diu-Scrip	Zide
Esidrix	
Hydro-Chlor	
HydroDiuril	
Hydromal	
Hydro-T	
Hydro-Z-50	

(Also available in generic form)

Type of Drug

Thiazide diuretic

Prescribed for

The initial treatment of hypertension. May be administered with other antihypertensive medications.

Cautions and Warnings

Do not take hydrochlorothiazide if you are allergic or sensitive to it, to other diuretics, or to sulfa drugs.

Although diuretics have been used to treat specific conditions in pregnancy, in general use by pregnant women should be avoided. Hydrochlorothiazide can cross the placental barrier and pass into the unborn child, creating the potential for problems. Diuretics are also found in the breast milk of nursing mothers.

Use hydrochlorothiazide with caution if you suffer from kidney or liver disease.

Hydrochlorothiazide may activate or worsen gout or lupus (systemic lupus erythematosus).

Hydrochlorothiazide will increase urination, so you should take the pills early in the day.

To avoid upset stomach, take the pills with food or milk.

Possible Side Effects

Hydrochlorothiazide may cause an electrolyte imbalance (potassium loss) in the body. *Signs of low potassium levels* are: dryness of the mouth; thirst; weakness; lethargy; drowsiness; restlessness; muscle pains or cramps; gout; muscle fatigue; decreased frequency of urination and amount of urine; abnormal heart rate; stomach upset (including nausea and vomiting).

To treat this, potassium supplements are available in the form of tablets, liquids, or powders; or your doctor may suggest increased consumption of potassium-rich foods such as bananas, citrus fruits, melons, and tomatoes.

Possible Adverse Effects

Loss of appetite; stomach upset; nausea; vomiting; cramping; diarrhea; constipation; dizziness; headache; tingling of the toes and fingers; restlessness; changes in blood composition; sensitivity to sunlight; rash; itching; fever; difficulty in breathing; allergic reactions; dizziness when rising quickly from a sitting or lying position; muscle spasms; weakness; blurred vision. Rare incidents of impotence have also been reported.

Drug Interactions

Hydrochlorothiazide may make the action of other blood-pressure-lowering drugs more effective. This is almost always a beneficial action, but your doctor may want to lower your dosage of the other antihypertensive drug.

The possibility of developing imbalances in body fluids and electrolytes is increased if you take certain medications—such as digitalis or adrenal corticosteroids—while you take hydrochlorothiazide.

If you are taking an oral antidiabetic drug and begin taking hydrochlorothiazide, the antidiabetic dose may have to be adjusted. Insulin requirements may also be affected.

Lithium carbonate should not be taken with diuretics because the combination may increase the risk of lithium toxicity.

If you are taking hydrochlorothiazide, avoid over-the-counter medications for the treatment of coughs, colds, and allergies, which may contain stimulants that raise your blood pressure. If you are unsure about which contain stimulants, ask your doctor or pharmacist.

Usual Dose

Initial dose: 50 to 100 mg. daily in single or divided doses.
Maintenance dose: 25 to 200 mg. daily.

Overdosage

Symptoms are fatigue, confusion, dizziness, nausea, lethargy, and coma. If you think you are experiencing an overdose, contact your doctor immediately, or go to a hospital emergency room. ALWAYS bring the medicine bottle with you.

Generic Name
Hydroflumethiazide

Brand Names

Diucardin
Saluron

Type of Drug

Thiazide diuretic

Prescribed for

The initial treatment of hypertension. May be administered with other antihypertensive medications.

Cautions and Warnings

Do not take hydroflumethiazide if you are allergic or sensitive to it, to other diuretics, or to sulfa drugs.

Although diuretics have been used to treat specific conditions in pregnancy, in general use by pregnant women should be avoided. Hydroflumethiazide can cross the placental barrier and pass into the unborn child, creating the potential for problems. Diuretics are also found in the breast milk of nursing mothers.

Use hydroflumethiazide with caution if you suffer from kidney or liver disease.

Hydroflumethiazide may activate or worsen gout or lupus (systemic lupus erythematosus).

Hydroflumethiazide will increase urination, so you should take it early in the day.

To avoid upset stomach, take the pills with food or milk.

Possible Side Effects

Hydroflumethiazide may cause an electrolyte imbalance (potassium loss) in the body. *Signs of low potassium levels* are: dryness of the mouth; thirst; weakness; lethargy; drowsiness; restlessness; muscle pains or cramps; gout; muscle fatigue; decreased frequency of urination and amount of urine; abnormal heart rate; stomach upset (including nausea and vomiting).

To treat this, potassium supplements are available in the form of tablets, liquids, or powders; or your doctor may suggest increased consumption of potassium-rich foods such as bananas, citrus fruits, melons, and tomatoes.

Possible Adverse Effects

Loss of appetite; stomach upset; nausea; vomiting; cramping; diarrhea; constipation; dizziness; headache; tingling of the toes and fingers; restlessness; changes in blood composition; sensitivity to sunlight; rash; itching; fever; difficulty in breathing; allergic reactions; dizziness when rising quickly from a sitting or lying position; muscle spasms; weakness; blurred vision. Rare incidents of impotence have also been reported.

Drug Interactions

Hydroflumethiazide may make the action of other blood-pressure-lowering drugs more effective. This is almost always a beneficial action, but your doctor may want to lower your dosage of the other antihypertensive drug.

The possibility of developing imbalances in body fluids and electrolytes is increased if you take certain medications—such as digitalis or adrenal corticosteroids—while you take hydroflumethiazide.

If you are taking an oral antidiabetic drug and begin taking hydroflumethiazide, the antidiabetic dose may have to be adjusted. Insulin requirements may also be affected.

Lithium carbonate should not be taken with diuretics because the combination may increase the risk of lithium toxicity.

If you are taking hydroflumethiazide, avoid over-the-counter medications for the treatment of coughs, colds, and allergies, which may contain stimulants that raise your blood pressure. If you are unsure about which contain stimulants, ask your doctor or pharmacist.

Usual Dose

Initial dose: 50 mg. twice daily.
Maintenance dose: 50 to 100 mg. daily.

Overdosage

Symptoms are fatigue, confusion, dizziness, nausea, lethargy, and coma. If you think you are experiencing an overdose, contact your doctor immediately, or go to a hospital emergency room. ALWAYS bring the medicine bottle with you.

Generic Name
Indapamide

Brand Name

Lozol

Type of Drug

Indoline

Prescribed for

The treatment of hypertension—either alone or with other antihypertensive medications.

Cautions and Warnings

Use with caution if you suffer from kidney or liver disease.

Indapamide can result in electrolyte and mineral imbalances (i.e., potassium loss). The warning signs for these imbalances are dry mouth; thirst; fatigue; weakness; muscle pains or cramps; stomach problems; drowsiness; restlessness; rapid heartbeat; nausea; vomiting; decreases in the amount of urine or frequency of urination; dizziness. Notify your doctor if you experience any of these symptoms.

Insulin requirements may have to be altered while taking indapamide.

Indapamide may initiate or worsen conditions of lupus (systemic lupus erythematosus) or gout.

Indapamide will increase your urination, so you should take it early in the day.

Pregnant women should only use this drug when the potential benefits clearly outweigh the unknown potential hazards to the fetus.

Safety for use by nursing mothers has not been established; therefore, mothers should not breastfeed while taking this drug.

Possible Side Effects

Headache; tingling in the arms or feet; nervousness; tension; irritability; constipation; light-headedness; insomnia; depression; blurred vision.

Possible Adverse Effects

Rash; hives; decreased sex drive or impotence; loss of appetite; irregular heartbeat.

Drug Interactions

Lithium should not be given with indapamide because this combination will increase the chances of lithium toxicity.

Indapamide may decrease the effectiveness of norepinephrine.

Usual Dose

Initial dose: 2.5 mg. once daily.
Maintenance dose: 2.5 to 5 mg. once daily.

Overdosage

The symptoms are nausea, vomiting, weakness, and stomach problems. A severe overdose may result in extremely low blood pressure and slow respiration. If you think you are experiencing an overdose, call your doctor immediately, or go to a hospital emergency room. ALWAYS bring the medicine bottle with you.

Brand Name
Inderide

Ingredients

Hydrochlorothiazide
Propranolol Hydrochloride

Type of Drug

Antihypertensive medication combining a diuretic (hydrochlorothiazide) with a beta blocker (propranolol hydrochloride).

Prescribed for

The treatment of hypertension when the initial diuretic treatment does not provide satisfactory results.

Cautions and Warnings

Do not take Inderide if you are allergic to either of its active ingredients or to sulfa drugs. If you have a history of heart failure, asthma, or upper respiratory disease, inderide may aggravate the situation.

Do not stop taking inderide unless your doctor tells you to do so.

If you develop a rash, severe muscle pains, or difficulty in breathing, call your doctor.

Avoid any over-the-counter drugs containing stimulants. If you are unsure which ones to avoid, ask your doctor or pharmacist.

Possible Side Effects

May decrease the heart rate or aggravate heart failure or some other heart diseases; tingling in the hands or feet; light-headedness; depression; sleeplessness; weakness; tiredness; feeling of not caring; hallucinations; visual disturbances; disorientation; loss of short-term memory; nausea; vomiting; upset stomach; cramps; diarrhea; constipation; allergic reactions including sore throat, rash, and fever. Inderide can also cause adverse effects on the blood.

Inderide can cause a lowering of body potassium (hypokalemia). The signs of this are: dryness of the mouth; weakness; thirst; lethargy; drowsiness; restlessness; muscle pains or cramps; muscle tiredness; low blood pressure; decreased frequency of urination. To treat this, potassium supplements are available in the form of tablets, liquids or powders; or your doctor may suggest increased consumption of potassium-rich foods such as bananas, citrus fruits, melons, or tomatoes.

Possible Adverse Effects

Loss of appetite; dizziness; headache; increased sensitivity to the sun; dizziness when rising quickly from a sitting or lying position; muscle spasms; loss of hearing (it comes back after inderide has been stopped).

Drug Interactions

Inderide may interact with reserpine and similar drugs to cause very low blood pressure, slowed heart rate, and dizziness.

Inderide may cause a need for the alteration of your daily dose of oral antidiabetic drug.

Inderide should not be taken with lithium drugs since there is an increased possibility of lithium toxicity. Inderide may interact with digitalis drugs to cause abnormal heart rhythms.

Usual Dose

Individualized to suit your needs.

Overdosage

Symptoms are fatigue, confusion, dizziness, nausea, lethargy, slowed heart rate, excessively low blood pressure, and coma.

If you think you are experiencing an overdose, contact your doctor immediately, or go to a hospital emergency room. ALWAYS bring the medicine bottle with you.

Generic Name
Methyclothiazide

Brand Names

Aquatensen
Enduron
Ethon
(Also available in generic form)

Type of Drug

Thiazide diuretic

Prescribed for

The initial treatment of hypertension. May be administered with other antihypertensive medications.

Cautions and Warnings

Do not take methyclothiazide if you are allergic or sensitive to it, to other diuretics, or to sulfa drugs.

Although diuretics have been used to treat specific conditions in pregnancy, in general use by pregnant women should be avoided. Methyclothiazide can cross the placental barrier and pass into the unborn child, creating the potential for problems. Diuretics are also found in the breast milk of nursing mothers.

Use methyclothiazide with caution if you suffer from kidney or liver disease.

Methyclothiazide may activate or worsen gout or lupus (systemic lupus erythematosus).

Methyclothiazide will increase urination, so you should take it early in the day.

To avoid upset stomach, take the pills with food or milk.

Possible Side Effects

Methyclothiazide may cause an electrolyte imbalance (potassium loss) in the body. *Signs of low potassium levels* are: dryness of the mouth; thirst; weakness; lethargy; drowsiness; restlessness; muscle pains or cramps; gout; muscle fatigue; decreased frequency of urination and amount of urine; abnormal heart rate; stomach upset (including nausea and vomiting).

To treat this, potassium supplements are available in the form of tablets, liquids, or powders; or your doctor may suggest increased consumption of potassium-rich foods such as bananas, citrus fruits, melons, and tomatoes.

Possible Adverse Effects

Loss of appetite; stomach upset; nausea; vomiting; cramping; diarrhea; constipation; dizziness; headache; tingling of the toes and fingers; restlessness; changes in blood composition; sensitivity to sunlight; rash; itching; fever; difficulty in breathing; allergic reactions; dizziness when rising quickly from a sitting or lying position; muscle spasms; weakness; blurred vision. Rare incidents of impotence have also been reported.

Drug Interactions

Methyclothiazide may make the action of other blood-pressure-lowering drugs more effective. This is almost always a beneficial action, but your doctor may want to lower your dosage of the other antihypertensive drug.

The possibility of developing imbalances in body fluids and electrolytes is increased if you take certain medications—such as digitalis or adrenal corticosteroids—while you take methyclothiazide.

If you are taking an oral antidiabetic drug and begin taking methyclothiazide, the antidiabetic dose may have to be adjusted. Insulin requirements may also be affected.

Lithium carbonate should not be taken with diuretics because the combination may increase the risk of lithium toxicity.

If you are taking methyclothiazide, avoid over-the-counter medications for the treatment of coughs, colds, and allergies, which may contain stimulants that raise your blood pressure. If you are unsure about which contain stimulants, ask your doctor or pharmacist.

Usual Dose

2.5 to 5 mg. once daily.

Overdosage

Symptoms are fatigue, confusion, dizziness, nausea, lethargy, and coma. If you think you are experiencing an overdose, contact your doctor immediately, or go to a hospital emergency room. ALWAYS bring the medicine bottle with you.

Generic Name
Methyldopa

Brand Name

Aldomet

Type of Drug

Antiadrenergic agent

Prescribed for

The treatment of hypertension—either alone or with a diuretic and/or other antihypertensive medications.

Cautions and Warnings

Do not take methyldopa if you have hepatitis or active cirrhosis, or if you have ever developed a sign or symptom of reaction to methyldopa.

Do not stop taking methyldopa unless directed to do so by your doctor.

Occasionally some people develop a tolerance to methyldopa (usually between the second and third months of therapy). This tolerance may require an adjustment in your antihypertensive medication.

Pregnant women should use methyldopa only if the potential benefits clearly outweigh the unknown potential hazards to the fetus.

Since methyldopa is found in breast milk, mothers should not breast-feed when taking this drug.

Contact your doctor immediately if you develop fever or experience any unexplained, prolonged general tiredness.

Possible Side Effects

Drowsiness during the first few weeks of therapy or when the dosage is increased. Headache or weakness are other possible side effects.

Possible Adverse Effects

Dizziness; light-headedness; tingling in the extremities; unusual muscle spasms; confusion; psychic disturbances (including nightmares, mild psychosis, or depression); changes in heart rate; chest pain; weight gain; retention of water; dizziness when rising suddenly from a sitting or reclining position; nausea; vomiting; constipation; diarrhea; dry mouth; sore and/or black tongue; stuffy nose; breast enlargement; lactation (in females); impotence or decreased sex drive; mild symptoms of arthritis; skin reactions.

Methyldopa can cause liver disorders: you may develop jaundice (yellowing of the skin and/or whites of the eyes), with or without fever, in the first 2 or 3 months of therapy. If you are taking methyldopa for the first time, be sure that your doctor checks your liver function, especially during the first 6 to 12 weeks of therapy. If your reactions are due to methyldopa, your temperature and/or liver abnormalities will return to normal as soon as the drug is discontinued.

Drug Interactions

Methyldopa may make the action of other blood-pressure-lowering drugs more effective. This is almost always a beneficial action, but your doctor may want to lower your dosage of the other antihypertensive drug.

Avoid over-the-counter cough, cold, or allergy medications unless approved by your doctor or pharmacist.

Methyldopa may impair the effectiveness of oral antidiabetic drugs such as tolbutamide, resulting in increased low blood-sugar levels.

If given together with phenoxybenzamine, inability to control one's bladder (urinary incontinence) may result.

The combination of methyldopa and lithium may cause symptoms of lithium overdose, even though blood levels of lithium do not change.

Methyldopa, when given in combination with haloperidol, may produce irritability, aggressiveness, assaultive behavior, or other psychiatric disturbances.

Usual Dose

Initial dose: 250 mg. tablet 2 to 3 times daily for the first 2 days.

Maintenance dose: 500 mg. to 2 grams in divided daily doses.

Overdosage

No data available.

Generic Name

Metolazone

Brand Names

Diulo
Zaroxolyn

Type of Drug

Thiazidelike diuretic

Prescribed for

The initial treatment of hypertension. May be administered with other antihypertensive medications.

Cautions and Warnings

Do not take metolazone if you are allergic or sensitive to it, or to other diuretics, or to sulfa drugs.

Although diuretics have been used to treat specific conditions in pregnancy, in general use by pregnant women should be avoided. Metolazone can cross the placental barrier and pass into the unborn child, creating the potential for problems. Diuretics are also found in the breast milk of nursing mothers.

Use metolazone with caution if you suffer from kidney or liver disease.

Metolazone may activate or worsen gout or lupus (systemic lupus erythematosus).

Metolazone will increase urination, so you should take it early in the day.

To avoid upset stomach, take the pills with food or milk.

Possible Side Effects

Metolazone may cause an electrolyte imbalance (potassium loss) in the body. *Signs of low potassium levels* are: dryness of the mouth; thirst; weakness; lethargy; drowsiness; restlessness; muscle pains or cramps; gout; muscle fatigue; decreased frequency of urination and amount of urine; abnormal heart rate; stomach upset (including nausea and vomiting).

To treat this, potassium supplements are available in the form of tablets, liquids, or powders; or your doctor may suggest increased consumption of potassium-rich foods such as bananas, citrus fruits, melons, and tomatoes.

Possible Adverse Effects

Loss of appetite; stomach upset; nausea; vomiting; cramping; diarrhea; constipation; dizziness; headache; tingling of the toes and fingers; restlessness; changes in blood composition; sensitivity to sunlight; rash; itching; fever; difficulty in breathing; allergic reactions; dizziness when rising quickly from a sitting or lying position; muscle spasms; weakness; blurred vision. Rare incidents of impotence have also been reported.

Drug Interactions

Metolazone may make the action of other blood-pressure-lowering drugs more effective. This is almost always a beneficial action, but your doctor may want to lower your dosage of the other antihypertensive drug.

The possibility of developing imbalances in body fluids and electrolytes is increased if you take certain medications—such as digitalis or adrenal corticosteroids—while you take metolazone.

If you are taking an oral antidiabetic drug and begin taking metolazone, the antidiabetic dose may have to be adjusted. Insulin requirements may also be affected.

Lithium carbonate should not be taken with diuretics because the combination may increase the risk of lithium toxicity.

If you are taking metolazone, avoid over-the-counter medications for the treatment of coughs, colds, and allergies, which may contain stimulants that raise your blood pressure. If you are unsure about which products contain stimulants, ask your doctor or pharmacist.

Usual Dose

2.5 to 5 mg. once daily.

Overdosage

Symptoms are fatigue, confusion, dizziness, nausea, lethargy, and coma. If you think you are experiencing an overdose, contact your doctor immediately, or go to a hospital emergency room. ALWAYS bring the medicine bottle with you.

Generic Name
Metoprolol Tartrate

Brand Name

Lopressor

Type of Drug

Beta blocker

Prescribed for

The treatment of hypertension as the first step or when diuretics have failed to lower blood pressure. Frequently, beta blockers are prescribed in combination with other antihypertensive medications.

Cautions and Warnings

Notify your doctor if you experience sore throat; fever; difficulty in breathing; night cough; swelling of the arms or legs; slow pulse rate; dizziness; light-headedness; confusion; depression; skin rash; unusual bleeding or bruising.

Metoprolol tartrate should be used with care if you have a history of asthma or upper respiratory disease, seasonal allergies, or other respiratory conditions. These conditions may be worsened by metoprolol tartrate. Metoprolol tartrate may also aggravate congestive heart failure.

Do not take metoprolol tartrate if you are allergic to any other beta blocker.

Diabetics should use this drug with caution because it may mask signs of hypoglycemia or alter blood glucose levels.

Do NOT suddenly stop taking metoprolol tartrate. Sudden cessation may result in angina (chest pain) or a worsening of any thyroid problems. Withdrawal from metoprolol tartrate should be gradual and under a doctor's direction.

Metoprolol tartrate may mask signs of hyperthyroidism and give the false impression that a thyroid condition is improving.

Use metoprolol tartrate with caution if you suffer from kidney or liver disease.

Safety for use during pregnancy has not been established. Pregnant women should use this drug only if the potential benefits clearly outweigh the unknown potential hazards to the fetus.

Mothers should not breast-feed while taking metoprolol tartrate.

Metoprolol tartrate may make you tired, so use caution when driving or performing tasks that require concentration.

Possible Side Effects

Light-headedness; insomnia; weakness; fatigue; visual disturbances; hallucinations; disorientation; short-term memory loss; nausea; vomiting; stomach upset; abdominal cramping and diarrhea; constipation.

Possible Adverse Effects

Decreased heart rate; excessively low blood pressure; tingling in the extremities; fainting; difficulty in breathing; chest pain.

Drug Interactions

Do not take metoprolol tartrate in combination with MAO inhibitors (there should be a 2-week period between the cessation of MAO inhibitor therapy and the start of beta-blocker treatment).

Metoprolol tartrate may increase the effectiveness of insulin or oral antidiabetic drugs. If you are diabetic, discuss the situation with your doctor; probably he/she will reduce the dosage of your antidiabetic medication.

Metoprolol tartrate may alter the effectiveness of digitalis on your heart. The digitalis dosage may have to be changed.

Metoprolol tartrate may make the action of other blood-pressure-lowering drugs more effective. This is almost always a beneficial action, but your doctor may want to lower your dosage of the other antihypertensive drug.

While taking this drug, do not use over-the-counter cough, cold, or allergy medications unless these products have been approved by your doctor or pharmacist.

The effects of metoprolol tartrate may be reversed by isoproterenol, norepinephrine, dopamine, or dobutamine.

Usual Dose

Initial dose: 100 mg. daily.
Maintenance dose: 100 to 450 mg. daily.

Overdosage

Symptoms are slowed heart rate, heart failure, excessively low blood pressure, and spasms of the bronchial muscles, which make it difficult to breathe. If you think you are experiencing an overdose, contact your doctor immediately, or go to a hospital emergency room. ALWAYS bring the medicine bottle with you.

Generic Name
Minoxidil

Brand Name

Loniten

Type of Drug

Vasodilator

Prescribed for

The treatment of severe hypertension that has not responded to other forms of drug treatment. NOT recommended for mild hypertension.

Cautions and Warnings

Minoxidil should not be used by people who have pheochromocytoma, a rare tumor in which extra body stimulants (catecholamines) are made.

Minoxidil may cause excess accumulation of water and sodium in the body, leading to heart failure. It also increases heart rate. To avoid these side effects, minoxidil should be taken with other drugs, such as a diuretic and a beta blocker.

Minoxidil should be avoided by pregnant women and nursing mothers unless absolutely necessary. The effect of this drug on fetuses is not known.

The effect of minoxidil on people who have suffered a recent (one month previous) heart attack has not been carefully studied.

Use minoxidil with caution if you suffer from kidney disease.

Notify your doctor if you experience rapid heartbeat; weight gain greater than 5 pounds; swelling of the hands, feet, face, or abdomen; difficulty in breathing; chest, arm, or shoulder pains; severe indigestion; dizziness; fainting.

Possible Side Effects

Swelling of the hands, face, feet, or stomach.

Most people who take minoxidil (80 percent) experience thickening, elongation, and darkening of body hair within 3 to 6 weeks after starting the drug. It is usually first noticed on the temples, between the eyebrows, between the eyebrows and hairline, or on the upper cheek. Later it may extend to the arms, back, legs, and scalp. (If this excessive hair growth bothers you, ask your doctor to recommend a medically safe hair remover.) This side effect ends when the drug is stopped, and hair returns to normal within 1 to 6 months.

Possible Adverse Effects

Nausea; vomiting; breast tenderness; fatigue; headache; darkening of the skin.

Drug Interactions

Minoxidil may interact with guanethidine to produce extreme dizziness.

Usual Dose

Initial dose: 5 mg. once daily.
Maintenance dose: 10 to 40 mg. daily.

Overdosage

Symptoms may include fainting, extreme dizziness, or coma. If you think you are experiencing an overdose, contact your doctor immediately, or go to a hospital emergency room. ALWAYS bring the medicine bottle with you.

Brand Name
Moduretic

Ingredients

Amiloride Hydrochloride
Hydrochlorothiazide

Type of Drug

Antihypertensive medication combining a potassium-sparing diuretic (amiloride hydrochloride) with a thiazide diuretic (hydrochlorothiazide).

Prescribed for

The treatment of hypertension when it is necessary to counteract the potassium loss caused by
diuretics.

Cautions and Warnings

Do not take Moduretic if you suffer from diabetes or kidney disease or are allergic to either of the
ingredients or to sulfa drugs. This drug may cause
abnormally high blood potassium levels. Since too
much potassium in your blood can be fatal, your
doctor should test your blood potassium levels
periodically. Moduretic should be used by pregnant women or nursing mothers only if absolutely
necessary.

Moduretic can affect your concentration. Do not
drive or operate machinery while taking it.

Possible Side Effects

Headache; weakness; tiredness; dizziness; difficulty in breathing; abnormal heart rhythms; nausea;
loss of appetite; diarrhea; stomach and abdominal pains; paradoxical decrease in blood potassium;
rash; itching; leg pains.

Possible Adverse Effects

Feeling sick; chest and back pain; heart palpitations; dizziness when rising from a sitting or lying
position; angina pain; constipation; stomach
bleeding; stomach upset; appetite changes; feeling of being bloated; hiccups; thirst; vomiting;
stomach gas; gout; dehydration; flushing; muscle cramps or spasms; joint pain; tingling in the
arms or legs; feeling of numbness; stupor; sleeplessness; nervousness; depression; sleepiness;

confusion; visual disturbances; bad taste in the mouth; stuffy nose; sexual impotence; urinary difficulties; dryness of the mouth; adverse effects on the blood system; fever; shock; allergic reactions; jaundice; liver damage; sugar in the blood or urine; unusual sensitivity to the sun; restlessness.

Drug Interactions

Moduretic may make the action of other blood-pressure-lowering drugs more effective. This is almost always a beneficial action, but your doctor may want to lower your dosage of the other antihypertensive drug.

The possibility of developing imbalances in body fluids (electrolytes) is increased if you take other medications—such as digitalis or adrenal corticosteroids—while you are taking Moduretic.

If you are taking an oral antidiabetic drug and begin taking Moduretic, the antidiabetic dose may have to be altered.

Lithium carbonate should not be taken with Moduretic because the combination may increase the risk of lithium toxicity.

Avoid over-the-counter cough, cold, or allergy remedies containing stimulant drugs that can aggravate your condition.

Moduretic may interfere with oral blood-thinning drugs (such as Warfarin) by making the blood more concentrated (thicker).

Usual Dose

1 to 2 tablets daily.

Overdosage

Signs are tingling in the arms or legs; weakness;

fatigue; slow heartbeat; sickly feeling; dryness of the mouth; lethargy; restlessness; muscle pains or cramps; low blood pressure; rapid heartbeat; urinary difficulty; nausea; vomiting. If you think you are experiencing an overdose, contact your doctor immediately, or go to a hospital emergency room. ALWAYS bring the medicine bottle with you.

Generic Name
Nadolol

Brand Name

Corgard

Type of Drug

Beta blocker

Prescribed for

The treatment of hypertension as the first step or when diuretics have failed to lower blood pressure. Frequently, beta blockers are prescribed in combination with other antihypertensive medications.

Cautions and Warnings

Notify your doctor if you experience sore throat; fever; difficulty in breathing; night cough; swelling of the arms or legs; slow pulse rate; dizziness; light-headedness; confusion; depression; skin rash; unusual bleeding or bruising.

Nadolol should be used with care if you have a history of asthma or upper respiratory disease, seasonal allergies, or other respiratory conditions. These conditions may be worsened by nadolol.

Nadolol may also aggravate congestive heart failure.

Do not take nadolol if you are allergic to any other beta blocker.

Diabetics should use nadolol with caution because it may mask signs of hypoglycemia or alter blood glucose levels.

Do NOT suddenly stop taking nadolol. Sudden cessation may result in angina (chest pain) or a worsening of any thyroid problems. Withdrawal from nadolol should be gradual and under a doctor's direction.

Nadolol may mask signs of hyperthyroidism and give the false impression that a thyroid condition is improving.

Use nadolol with caution if you suffer from kidney or liver disease.

Safety for use during pregnancy has not been established. Pregnant women should use this drug only if the potential benefits clearly outweigh the unknown potential hazards to the fetus.

Mothers should not breast-feed while taking nadolol.

Nadolol may make you tired, so use caution when driving or performing tasks that require concentration.

Possible Side Effects

Light-headedness; insomnia; weakness; fatigue; visual disturbances; hallucinations; disorientation; short-term memory loss; nausea; vomiting; stomach upset; abdominal cramping and diarrhea; constipation.

Possible Adverse Effects

Decreased heart rate; excessively low blood pressure; tingling in the extremities; fainting; difficulty in breathing; chest pain.

Drug Interactions

Do not take nadolol in combination with MAO inhibitors (there should be a 2-week period between the cessation of MAO inhibitor therapy and the start of beta-blocker treatment).

Nadolol may increase the effectiveness of insulin or oral antidiabetic drugs. If you are diabetic, discuss the situation with your doctor; probably he/she will reduce the dosage of your antidiabetic medication.

Nadolol may alter the effectiveness of digitalis on your heart. The digitalis dosage may have to be changed.

Nadolol may make the action of other blood-pressure-lowering drugs more effective. This is almost always a beneficial action, but your doctor may want to lower your dosage of the other antihypertensive drug.

While taking nadolol do not use over-the-counter cough, cold, or allergy medications unless these products have been approved by your doctor or pharmacist.

The effects of nadolol may be reversed by isoproterenol, norepinephrine, dopamine, or dobutamine.

Usual Dose

Initial dose: 40 mg. once daily.
Maintenance dose: 80 to 320 mg. once daily.

Overdosage

Symptoms are slowed heart rate, heart failure, excessively low blood pressure, and spasms of the bronchial muscles, which make it difficult to breathe. If you think you are experiencing an overdose, contact your doctor immediately, or go to a hospital emergency room. ALWAYS bring the medicine bottle with you.

Generic Name
Pindolol

Brand Name

Visken

Type of Drug

Beta blocker

Prescribed for

The treatment of hypertension as the first step or when diuretics have failed to lower blood pressure. Frequently, beta blockers are prescribed in combination with other antihypertensive medications.

Cautions and Warnings

Notify your doctor if you experience sore throat; fever; difficulty in breathing; night cough; swelling of the arms or legs; slow pulse rate; dizziness; light-headedness; confusion; depression; skin rash; unusual bleeding or bruising.

Pindolol should be used with care if you have a history of asthma or upper respiratory disease, seasonal allergies, or other respiratory conditions. These conditions may be worsened by pindolol. Pindolol may also aggravate congestive heart failure.

Do not take pindolol if you are allergic to any other beta blocker.

Diabetics should use this drug with caution because it may mask signs of hypoglycemia or alter blood glucose levels.

Do NOT suddenly stop taking pindolol. Sudden cessation may result in angina (chest pain) or a worsening of any thyroid problems. Withdrawal from pindolol should be gradual and under a doctor's direction.

Pindolol may mask signs of hyperthyroidism and give the false impression that a thyroid condition is improving.

Use pindolol with caution if you suffer from kidney or liver disease.

Safety for use during pregnancy has not been established. Pregnant women should use pindolol only if the potential benefits clearly outweigh the unknown potential hazards to the fetus.

Mothers should not breast-feed while taking pindolol.

Pindolol may make you tired, so use caution when driving or performing tasks that require concentration.

Possible Side Effects

Light-headedness; insomnia; weakness; fatigue; visual disturbances; hallucinations; disorientation; short-term memory loss; nausea; vomiting; stomach upset; abdominal cramping and diarrhea; constipation.

Possible Adverse Effects

Decreased heart rate; excessively low blood pressure; tingling in the extremities; fainting; difficulty in breathing; chest pain.

Drug Interactions

Do not take pindolol in combination with MAO

inhibitors (there should be a 2-week period between the cessation of MAO inhibitor therapy and the start of beta-blocker treatment).

Pindolol may increase the effectiveness of insulin or oral antidiabetic drugs. If you are diabetic, discuss the situation with your doctor; probably he/she will reduce the dosage of your antidiabetic medication.

This drug may alter the effectiveness of digitalis on your heart. The digitalis dosage may have to be changed.

Pindolol may make the action of other blood-pressure-lowering drugs more effective. This is almost always a beneficial action, but your doctor may want to lower your dosage of the other antihypertensive drug.

While taking pindolol, do not use over-the-counter cough, cold, or allergy medications unless these products have been approved by your doctor or pharmacist.

The effects of pindolol may be reversed by isoproterenol, norepinephrine, dopamine, or dobutamine.

Usual Dose

Initial dose: 10 mg. twice daily.
Maintenance dose: 10 to 60 mg. daily.

Overdosage

Symptoms are slowed heart rate, heart failure, excessively low blood pressure, and spasms of the bronchial muscles, which make it difficult to breathe. If you think you are experiencing an overdose, contact your doctor immediately, or go to a hospital emergency room. ALWAYS bring the medicine bottle with you.

Generic Name
Polythiazide

Brand Name

Renese

Type of Drug

Thiazide diuretic

Prescribed for

The initial treatment of hypertension. May be administered with other antihypertensive medications.

Cautions and Warnings

Do not take polythiazide if you are allergic or sensitive to it, to other diuretics, or to sulfa drugs.

Although diuretics have been used to treat specific conditions in pregnancy, in general use by pregnant women should be avoided. Polythiazide can cross the placental barrier and pass into the unborn child, creating the potential for problems. Diuretics are also found in the breast milk of nursing mothers.

Use polythiazide with caution if you suffer from kidney or liver disease.

Polythiazide may activate or worsen gout or lupus (systemic lupus erythematosus).

Polythiazide will increase urination, so you should take it early in the day.

To avoid upset stomach, take the pills with food or milk.

Possible Side Effects

Polythiazide may cause an electrolyte imbalance

(potassium loss) in the body. *Signs of low potassium levels* are: dryness of the mouth; thirst; weakness; lethargy; drowsiness; restlessness; muscle pains or cramps; gout; muscle fatigue; decreased frequency of urination and amount of urine; abnormal heart rate; stomach upset (including nausea and vomiting).

To treat this, potassium supplements are available in the form of tablets, liquids, or powders; or your doctor may suggest increased consumption of potassium-rich foods such as bananas, citrus fruits, melons, and tomatoes.

Possible Adverse Effects

Loss of appetite; stomach upset; nausea; vomiting; cramping; diarrhea; constipation; dizziness; headache; tingling of the toes and fingers; restlessness; changes in blood composition; sensitivity to sunlight; rash; itching; fever; difficulty in breathing; allergic reactions; dizziness when rising quickly from a sitting or lying position; muscle spasms; weakness; blurred vision. Rare incidents of impotence have also been reported.

Drug Interactions

Polythiazide may make the action of other blood-pressure-lowering drugs more effective. This is almost always a beneficial action, but your doctor may want to lower your dosage of the other antihypertensive drug.

The possibility of developing imbalances in body fluids and electrolytes is increased if you take certain medications—such as digitalis or adrenal corticosteroids—while you take polythiazide.

If you are taking an oral antidiabetic drug and begin taking polythiazide, the antidiabetic dose may have to be adjusted. Insulin requirements may also be affected.

Lithium carbonate should not be taken with diuretics because the combination may increase the risk of lithium toxicity.

If you are taking polythiazide, avoid over-the-counter medications for the treatment of coughs, colds, and allergies, which may contain stimulants that raise your blood pressure. If you are unsure about which contain stimulants, ask your doctor or pharmacist.

Usual Dose

Initial dose: 2 to 4 mg. daily.
Maintenance dose: adjusted to suit your needs.

Overdosage

Symptoms are fatigue, confusion, dizziness, nausea, lethargy, and coma. If you think you are experiencing an overdose, contact your doctor immediately, or go to a hospital emergency room. ALWAYS bring the medicine bottle with you.

Generic Name
Potassium Chloride

Brand Name

Oral Tablets

Kaon-Cl (wax matrix)
Kao-Nor
Klotrix (wax matrix)
K-Forte
K-Tab (wax matrix)
Micro-K

Osto-K
Slow-K (wax matrix)
(Also available in generic form)

Effervescent tablets

Kaochlor-Eff
K-Lyte/Cl
Keff
Klorvess
K-Lyte

Powders

Kato
K-Lor
Klor-Con
Klorvess Granules
K-Lyte/Cl
Kay Ciel
Kolyum
Potage

Type of Drug

Potassium supplement

Prescribed for

Counteraction of the potassium loss caused by diuretics.

Cautions and Warnings

Potassium replacement should always be monitored and controlled by your doctor. Potassium chloride tablets have produced ulceration in some patients with compression of the esophagus. Potassium chloride supplements for these patients should be given in liquid form. Potassium chloride tablets have been reported to cause ulcers of the small bowel, leading to hemorrhage, obstruction, and/or perforation.

Do not take potassium chloride supplements if you are dehydrated or experiencing muscle cramps due to excessive sun exposure. The drug should be used with caution in patients who have kidney and/or heart disease.

Directions for taking potassium chloride supplements should be followed closely. Effervescent tablets and potassium chloride supplement powders should be dissolved completely. Tablets should be swallowed whole, not chewed or crushed.

Possible Side Effects

Nausea; vomiting; diarrhea; and abdominal discomfort.

Possible Adverse Effects

Less common side effects are: tingling of hands and feet; listlessness; mental confusion; weakness and heaviness of legs; decreased blood pressure and/or heart rhythm changes.

Drug Interactions

Potassium chloride supplements should not be taken with spironolactone, triamterene, or combinations of these drugs, as potassium chloride toxicity may occur.

Usual Dose

As regulated by your doctor.

Overdosage

Potassium chloride toxicity, or overdose, is extremely rare. Toxicity can occur when high doses of potassium chloride supplements are taken in combination with foods high in potassium chloride.

Overdose symptoms include weakness, difficulty in moving hands or legs, confusion, low blood pressure, irregular heart rhythms, and heart attack. If you think you are experiencing an overdose, contact your doctor immediately, or go to a hospital emergency room. ALWAYS bring the medicine bottle with you.

Generic Name
Prazosin Hydrochloride

Brand Name

Minipress

Type of Drug

Vasodilator

Prescribed for

The treatment of hypertension—either alone or with other antihypertensive medications.

Cautions and Warnings

Prazosin hydrochloride can cause dizziness and fainting. Most often, this occurs when one rises suddenly from a sitting or reclining position. Avoid sudden changes in posture to minimize this dizziness.

Because of the possibility of fainting and dizziness, special care must be observed when taking the first dose of prazosin hydrochloride. It is recommended that you avoid driving or performing tasks that require concentration for at least 4 hours after taking your first dose.

Do not stop taking prazosin hydrochloride unless directed to do so by your doctor.

Avoid cough, cold, and allergy remedies unless they have been approved by your doctor or pharmacist.

Pregnant women and nursing mothers should avoid prazosin hydrochloride unless absolutely necessary.

Possible Side Effects

Dizziness; headache; drowsiness; lack of energy; weakness; palpitations; nausea.

Possible Adverse Effects

Vomiting; diarrhea; constipation; stomach upset or pain; unusual swelling in the arms or legs; shortness of breath; fainting; rapid heart rate, increased chest pain (angina); nervousness; depression; tingling in the hands or feet; rash; itching; frequent urination; poor urinary control; sexual impotence; blurred vision; redness of the eyes; ringing or buzzing in the ears; dry mouth; stuffy nose; sweating.

Drug Interactions

Prazosin hydrochloride combined with nitroglycerin may cause fainting.

Usual Dose

Initial dose: 1 mg. 2 or 3 times daily.
Maintenance dose: 6 to 15 mg. in divided daily doses.

Overdosage

Symptoms may include fainting, dizziness, or coma. If you think you are experiencing an overdose, contact your doctor immediately, or go to a hospital emergency room. ALWAYS bring the medicine bottle with you.

Generic Name
Propranolol Hydrochloride

Brand Name

Inderal

Type of Drug

Beta blocker

Prescribed for

The treatment of hypertension as the first step or when diuretics have failed to lower blood pressure. Frequently, beta blockers are prescribed in combination with other antihypertensive medications.

Cautions and Warnings

Notify your doctor if you experience sore throat; fever; difficulty in breathing; night cough; swelling of the arms or legs; slow pulse rate; dizziness;

light-headedness; confusion; depression; skin rash; unusual bleeding or bruising.

Propranolol hydrochloride should be used with care if you have a history of asthma or upper respiratory disease, seasonal allergies, or other respiratory conditions. These conditions may be worsened by propranolol hydrochloride. Propranolol hydrochloride may also aggravate congestive heart failure.

Do not take propranolol hydrochloride if you are allergic to any other beta blocker.

Diabetics should use propranolol hydrochloride with caution because it may mask signs of hypoglycemia or alter blood glucose levels.

Do NOT suddenly stop taking propranolol hydrochloride. Sudden cessation may result in angina (chest pain) or a worsening of any thyroid problems. Withdrawal from propranolol hdyrochloride should be gradual and under a doctor's direction.

Propranolol hydrochloride may mask signs of hyperthyroidism and give the false impression that a thyroid condition is improving.

Use propranolol hydrochloride with caution if you suffer from kidney or liver disease.

Safety for use during pregnancy has not been established. Pregnant women should use propranolol hydrochloride only if the potential benefits clearly outweigh the unknown potential hazards to the fetus.

Mothers should not breast-feed while taking propranolol hydrochloride.

Propranolol hydrochloride may make you tired, so use caution when driving or performing tasks that require concentration.

Possible Side Effects

Light-headedness; insomnia; weakness; fatigue;

visual disturbances; hallucinations; disorientation; short-term memory loss; nausea; vomiting; stomach upset; abdominal cramping and diarrhea; constipation.

Possible Adverse Effects

Decreased heart rate; excessively low blood pressure; tingling in the extremities; fainting; difficulty in breathing; chest pain.

Occasionally, propranolol hydrochloride may cause emotional instability or unusual personality changes. Contact your doctor if you experience these symptoms.

Drug Interactions

Do not take propranolol hydrochloride in combination with MAO inhibitors (there should be a 2-week period between the cessation of MAO inhibitor therapy and the start of beta-blocker treatment).

Propranolol hydrochloride may increase the effectiveness of insulin or oral antidiabetic drugs. If you are diabetic, discuss the situation with your doctor; probably he/she will reduce the dosage of your antidiabetic medication.

Propranolol hydrochloride may alter the effectiveness of digitalis on your heart. The digitalis dosage may have to be changed.

Propranolol hydrochloride may make the action of other blood-pressure-lowering drugs more effective. This is almost always a beneficial action, but your doctor may want to lower your dosage of the other antihypertensive drug.

While taking propranolol hydrochloride do not use over-the-counter cough, cold, or allergy medications unless these products have been approved by your doctor or pharmacist.

The effects of propranolol hydrochloride may be reversed by isoproterenol, norepinephrine, dopamine, or dobutamine.

Indomethacin may limit the effectiveness of propranolol hydrochloride.

Usual Dose

Initial dose: 40 mg. twice daily.
Maintenance dose: 120 to 640 mg. daily.

Overdosage

Symptoms are slowed heart rate, heart failure, excessively low blood pressure, and spasms of the bronchial muscles, which make it difficult to breathe. If you think you are experiencing an overdose, contact your doctor immediately, or go to a hospital emergency room. ALWAYS bring the medicine bottle with you.

Generic Name
Quinethazone

Brand Name

Hydromox

Type of Drug

Thiazide diuretic

Prescribed for

The initial treatment of hypertension. May be administered with other antihypertensive medications.

Cautions and Warnings

Do not take quinethazone if you are allergic or sensitive to it, to other diuretics, or to sulfa drugs.

Although diuretics have been used to treat specific conditions in pregnancy, in general use by pregnant women should be avoided. Quinethazone can cross the placental barrier and pass into the unborn child, creating the potential for problems. Diuretics are also found in the breast milk of nursing mothers.

Use quinethazone with caution if you suffer from kidney or liver disease.

Quinethazone may activate or worsen gout or lupus (systemic lupus erythematosus).

Quinethazone will increase urination, so you should take it early in the day.

To avoid upset stomach, take the pills with food or milk.

Possible Side Effects

Quinethazone may cause an electrolyte imbalance (potassium loss) in the body. *Signs of low potassium levels* are: dryness of the mouth; thirst; weakness; lethargy; drowsiness; restlessness; muscle pains or cramps; gout; muscle fatigue; decreased frequency of urination and amount of urine; abnormal heart rate; stomach upset (including nausea and vomiting).

To treat this, potassium supplements are available in the form of tablets, liquids, or powders; or your doctor may suggest increased consumption of potassium-rich foods such as bananas, citrus fruits, melons, and tomatoes.

Possible Adverse Effects

Loss of appetite; stomach upset; nausea; vomiting; cramping; diarrhea; constipation; dizziness; headache; tingling of the toes and fingers; restlessness; changes in blood composition; sensitivity to sunlight; rash; itching; fever; difficulty in breathing; allergic reactions; dizziness when rising quickly from a sitting or lying position; muscle spasms; weakness; blurred vision. Rare incidents of impotence have also been reported.

Drug Interactions

Quinethazone may make the action of other blood-pressure-lowering drugs more effective. This is almost always a beneficial action, but your doctor may want to lower your dosage of the other antihypertensive drug.

The possibility of developing imbalances in body fluids and electrolytes is increased if you take certain medications—such as digitalis or adrenal corticosteroids—while you take quinethazone.

If you are taking an oral antidiabetic drug and begin taking quinethazone, the antidiabetic dose may have to be adjusted. Insulin requirements may also be affected.

Lithium carbonate should not be taken with diuretics because the combination may increase the risk of lithium toxicity.

If you are taking quinethazone, avoid over-the-counter medications for the treatment of coughs, colds, and allergies, which may contain stimulants that raise your blood pressure. If you are unsure about which contain stimulants, ask your doctor or pharmacist.

Usual Dose

Initial dose: 50 to 100 mg. once daily.
Maintenance dose: 50 to 200 mg. daily.

Overdosage

Symptoms are fatigue, confusion, dizziness, nausea, lethargy, and coma. If you think you are experiencing an overdose, contact your doctor immediately, or go to a hospital emergency room. ALWAYS bring the medicine bottle with you.

Generic Name
Rescinnamine

Brand Name

Moderil

Type of Drug

Antiadrenergic agent

Prescribed for

The treatment of hypertension—either alone or with other antihypertensive medications.

Cautions and Warnings

Do not stop taking rescinnamine unless directed to do so by your doctor.

Use with extreme caution if you suffer from depression, since rescinnamine may induce severe depression that may persist for several months after you stop taking it. Notify your doctor if you experience any changes in mood or sleep habits, or continual severe stomach pain.

Avoid cough, cold, or allergy medications except when they are approved by your doctor or pharmacist.

If dizziness occurs, avoid suddenly rising from a sitting or reclining position.

Pregnant women should use rescinnamine only when the potential benefits clearly outweigh the unknown potential hazards to the fetus.

Mothers should not breast-feed when taking rescinnamine.

Use rescinnamine with caution if you suffer from kidney or liver disease or have a history of peptic ulcers, ulcerative colitis, or gallstones.

This product may contain tartrazine, a substance found to cause allergic reactions, especially in people allergic to aspirin.

Possible Side Effects

Stuffy nose; dry mouth; dizziness; headache; breathing difficulties; impotence or decreased sex drive; muscle aches; weight gain; breast enlargement; lactation (in females).

Possible Adverse Effects

Nausea; vomiting; loss of appetite; diarrhea; stomach bleeding; chest pain; abnormal heart rhythms; swelling of hands or feet; depression; fainting; involuntary movements or twitching of the head and neck.

Drug Interactions

Digitalis and quinidine, when used with rescinnamine, may cause abnormal heart rhythms.

MAO inhibitors should be avoided or used with extreme caution.

Rescinnamine, when used with beta blockers, may result in extreme low blood pressure manifested by fainting, vertigo, or dizziness when suddenly rising from a sitting or reclining position.

Usual Dose

Initial dose: 0.5 mg. twice daily.
Maintenance dose: 0.25 to 0.5 mg. daily.

Overdosage

Symptoms are changes in consciousness rang-ing from dizziness to coma; diarrhea; difficulty in breathing; slow heartbeat; flushing of the skin; pupil constriction. If you think you are experienc-ing an overdose, call your doctor immediately, or go to a hospital emergency room. ALWAYS bring the medicine bottle with you.

Generic Name
Reserpine

Brand Names

Lemiserp	Serpanray
Rau-Sed	Serpasil
Releserp-5	Serpate
Reserjen	Zepine
Reserpoid	(Also available in generic form)
Sandril	
Serpalan	

Type of Drug

Antiadrenergic agent

Prescribed for

The treatment of hypertension—either alone or with other antihypertensive medications.

Cautions and Warnings

Do not stop taking reserpine unless directed to do so by your doctor.

Use with extreme caution if you suffer from depression, since reserpine may induce severe depression that may persist for several months after you stop taking it. Notify your doctor if you experience any changes in mood or sleep habits, or continual severe stomach pain.

Avoid cough, cold, or allergy medications except when they are approved by your doctor or pharmacist.

If dizziness occurs, avoid suddenly rising from a sitting or reclining position.

In some studies, use of reserpine by women was associated with a greater incidence of breast cancer. However, other studies failed to support these findings.

Pregnant women should use reserpine only when the potential benefits clearly outweigh the unknown potential hazards to the fetus.

Mothers should not breast-feed when taking reserpine.

Use reserpine with caution if you suffer from kidney or liver disease or have a history of peptic ulcers, ulcerative colitis, or gallstones.

This product may contain tartrazine, a substance found to cause allergic reactions, especially in people allergic to aspirin.

Possible Side Effects

Stuffy nose; dry mouth; dizziness; headache; breathing difficulties; impotence or decreased sex drive; muscle aches; weight gain; breast enlargement; lactation (in females).

Possible Adverse Effects

Nausea; vomiting; loss of appetite; diarrhea; stomach bleeding; chest pain; abnormal heart rhythms; swelling of hands or feet; depression; fainting; involuntary movements or twitching of the head and neck.

Drug Interactions

Digitalis and quinidine, when used with reserpine, may cause abnormal heart rhythms.

MAO inhibitors should be avoided or used with extreme caution.

Reserpine, when used with beta blockers, may result in extreme low blood pressure manifested by fainting, vertigo, or dizziness when suddenly rising from a sitting or reclining position.

Usual Dose

Initial dose: 0.5 mg. daily for 1 to 2 weeks.
Maintenance dose: 0.1 to 0.25 mg. daily.

Overdosage

Symptoms are changes in consciousness ranging from dizziness to coma; diarrhea; difficulty in breathing; slow heartbeat; flushing of the skin; pupil constriction. If you think you are experiencing an overdose, call your doctor immediately, or go to a hospital emergency room. ALWAYS bring the medicine bottle with you.

Brand Name
Ser-Ap-Es

Ingredients

Hydralazine Hydrochloride
Hydrochlorothiazide
Reserpine

Other Brand Names

Cam-ap-es	Ser-Hydra-Zine
Hydrap-ES	Tri-Hydroserpine
Hyserp	Unipres
R-HCTZ-H	
Ser-A-Gen	
Seralazide	

Type of Drug

Antihypertensive medication combining a vaso-dilator (hydralazine hydrochloride), a diuretic (hydrochlorothiazide), and an antiadrenergic agent (reserpine).

Prescribed for

The treatment of hypertension when the initial diuretic treatment does not provide satisfactory results.

Cautions and Warnings

Do not take Ser-Ap-Es tablets if you are sensitive or allergic to any of its ingredients or if you have a history of mental depression, active peptic ulcer, or ulcerative colitis. Long-term administration in large doses may produce symptoms similar to arthritis in a few patients. This usually resolves itself when you stop taking the drug. The recurrence of fever, chest pains, not feeling well, or other unexplained problems should be investigated further by your doctor.

It is important to eat a well-balanced diet or follow the special diet given to you by your doctor. You must take Ser-Ap-Es exactly as prescribed.

Slight stomach upset from Ser-Ap-Es tablets can be overcome by taking each dose with some food. If stomach pain continues or becomes severe, call your doctor.

Possible Side Effects

Headache; loss of appetite; vomiting; nausea; diarrhea; abnormal heart rate; chest pains; stomach upset; cramps; tingling in the arms and legs; restlessness; drowsiness; depression; nervousness; anxiety; nightmares; glaucoma; blood disorders; rash; itching; fever; difficulty in breathing; muscle spasms, weakness; high blood sugar; sugar in the urine; blurred vision; stuffy nose; dry mouth. Impotence and decreased sex drive have also been reported.

Possible Adverse Effects

Flushing of the skin, tearing of the eyes, conjunctivitis, disorientation, and anxiety are infrequent. Rarely, long-term users have developed symptoms of hepatitis.

Drug Interactions

Ser-Ap-Es tablets may interact with MAO inhibitor drugs, digitalis, or quinidine.

Ser-Ap-Es tablets will interact with drugs containing lithium, producing a higher incidence of adverse effects from the lithium products.

Avoid over-the-counter cough, cold, or allergy remedies that contain stimulant drugs, as these can counteract the antihypertensive medication.

Usual Dose

Individualized to suit your needs.

Overdosage

Symptoms are extreme lowering of blood pressure; rapid heartbeat; headache; generalized skin flushing; chest pains; poor heart rhythms. If you think you are experiencing an overdose, contact your doctor immediately, or go to a hospital emergency room. ALWAYS bring the medicine bottle with you.

Generic Name
Spironolactone

Brand Name

Aldactone
Spiractone
(Also available in generic form)

Type of Drug

Potassium-sparing diuretic

Prescribed for

The treatment of hypertension when it is important to avoid the potassium loss caused by other diuretics. May be used alone or in combination with other antihypertensive medications.

Cautions and Warnings

High blood levels of potassium associated with the use of spironolactone may cause weakness, lethargy, drowsiness, and muscle fatigue. Patients should be careful when driving or performing other tasks that require concentration.

Notify your doctor if you experience diarrhea; lethargy; thirst, headache; rash; menstrual abnormalities; deepening of the voice; breast enlargement.

Spironolactone should not be used if you have kidney failure or high blood levels of potassium.

While taking spironolactone, you should not take other potassium-sparing diuretics, potassium supplements, or foods rich in potassium (such as bananas, citrus fruits, melons, and tomatoes).

Spironolactone causes tumors when given in very high doses to laboratory rats.

If possible, pregnant or nursing women should not use spironolactone.

Possible Side Effects

Drowsiness; lethargy; headache; stomach upset; cramping and diarrhea; rash; mental confusion; fever; feeling of ill health.

Possible Adverse Effects

Enlargement of the breasts; inability to achieve or maintain an erection; irregular menstrual cycles or deepening of the voice (in females).

Drug Interactions

Spironolactone may make the action of other blood-pressure-lowering drugs more effective. This is almost always a beneficial action, but your doctor may want to lower your dosage of the other antihypertensive drug.

If you take spironolactone, do not use over-the-counter cough, cold, or allergy remedies unless your doctor or pharmacist has approved these products for your use.

Lithium should not be given with spironolactone, since there is a greater risk of reaching lithium toxicity.

The effectiveness of digitalis and oral anticoagulants may be lessened by spironolactone.

Usual Dose

Initial dose: 50 to 100 mg. daily.
Maintenance dose: adjusted to suit your needs.

Overdosage

No data available.

Generic Name
Timolol Maleate

Brand Name

Blocadren

Type of Drug

Beta blocker

Prescribed for

The treatment of hypertension as the first step or when diuretics have failed to lower blood pressure. Frequently, beta blockers are prescribed in combination with other antihypertensive medications.

Cautions and Warnings

Notify your doctor if you experience sore throat; fever; difficulty in breathing; night cough; swelling of the arms or legs; slow pulse rate; dizziness; light-headedness; confusion; depression; skin rash; unusual bleeding or bruising.

Timolol maleate should be used with care if you have a history of asthma or upper respiratory disease, seasonal allergies, or other respiratory conditions. These conditions may be worsened by timolol maleate. Timolol maleate may also aggravate congestive heart failure.

Do not take timolol maleate if you are allergic to any other beta blocker.

Diabetics should use timolol maleate with caution because it may mask signs of hypoglycemia or alter blood glucose levels.

Do NOT suddenly stop taking timolol maleate. Sudden cessation may result in angina (chest pain) or a worsening of any thyroid problems. Withdrawal from timolol maleate should be gradual and under a doctor's direction.

Timolol maleate may mask signs of hyperthyroidism and give the false impression that a thyroid condition is improving.

Use timolol maleate with caution if you suffer from kidney or liver disease.

Safety for use during pregnancy has not been established. Pregnant women should use timolol maleate only if the potential benefits clearly outweigh the unknown potential hazards to the fetus.

Mothers should not breast-feed while taking timolol maleate.

Timolol maleate may make you tired, so use caution when driving or performing tasks that require concentration.

Possible Side Effects

Light-headedness; insomnia; weakness; fatigue; visual disturbances; hallucinations; disorientation; short-term memory loss; nausea; vomiting; stomach upset; abdominal cramping and diarrhea; constipation.

Possible Adverse Effects

Decreased heart rate; excessively low blood pressure; tingling in the extremities; fainting; difficulty in breathing; chest pain.

Drug Interactions

Do not take timolol maleate in combination with MAO inhibitors (there should be a 2-week period between the cessation of MAO inhibitor therapy and the start of beta-blocker treatment).

Timolol maleate may increase the effectiveness of insulin or oral antidiabetic drugs. If you are diabetic, discuss the situation with your doctor, who will probably reduce the dosage of your antidiabetic medication.

Timolol maleate may alter the effectiveness of digitalis on your heart. The digitalis dosage may have to be changed.

Timolol maleate may make the action of other blood-pressure-lowering drugs more effective. This is almost always a beneficial action, but your doctor may want to lower your dosage of the other antihypertensive drug.

While taking timolol maleate, do not use over-the-counter cough, cold, or allergy medications unless these products have been approved by your doctor or pharmacist.

The effects of timolol maleate may be reversed

by isoproterenol, norepinephrine, dopamine, or dobutamine.

Usual Dose

Initial dose: 10 mg. twice daily.
Maintenance dose: 20 to 40 mg. daily.

Overdosage

Symptoms are slowed heart rate, heart failure, excessively low blood pressure, and spasms of the bronchial muscles, which make it difficult to breathe. If you think you are experiencing an overdose, contact your doctor immediately, or go to a hospital emergency room. ALWAYS bring the medicine bottle with you.

Generic Name
Triamterene

Brand Name

Dyrenium

Type of Drug

Potassium-sparing diuretic

Prescribed for

The treatment of hypertension when it is important to avoid the potassium loss caused by other diuretics. May be used alone or in combination with other antihypertensive medications.

Cautions and Warnings

Do not take triamterene if you suffer from kidney or liver disease.

Avoid prolonged exposure to sunlight, as photo-sensitive reactions (i.e., skin rashes, spots) may occur on exposed skin.

Pregnant women should not use this drug except when the potential benefits clearly outweigh the possibility of harm to the fetus.

Nursing mothers should not continue to breast-feed while taking triamterene, since this drug enters into the mother's milk.

While taking triamterene, avoid other potassium-sparing diuretics, potassium supplements, or foods rich in potassium (i.e., bananas, citrus fruits, melons, and tomatoes).

You should have blood tests on a regular basis to monitor your potassium level.

Possible Side Effects

Weakness; headache; dry mouth; rash; nausea; vomiting; stomach upset. Notify your doctor if these conditions become severe or occur frequently.

Possible Adverse Effects

Notify your doctor immediately if you experience fever, sore throat, mouth sores, unusual bleeding, or bruising.

Drug Interactions

Using triamterene with other antihypertensive drugs may result in the need to adjust the dosages of the other medications.

Using triamterene with digitalis may decrease the effectiveness of digitalis.

Use nonsteroidal anti-inflammatory drugs (e.g., indomethacin) with caution while taking triamterene.

In general, lithium should not be taken with diuretics because this combination may increase the possibility of lithium toxicity.

Usual Dose

Initial dose: 100 mg. twice daily (after meals).
Maintenance dose: adjusted to suit your needs.

Overdosage

Symptoms are nausea, vomiting, weakness. If you think you are experiencing an overdose, contact your doctor immediately, or go to a hospital emergency room. ALWAYS bring the medicine bottle with you.

Generic Name
Trichlormethiazide

Brand Names

Aquazide
Diurese
Metahydrin
Mono-Press
Naqua
Niazide
Trichlorex
(Also available in generic form)

Type of Drug

Thiazide diuretic

Prescribed for

The initial treatment of hypertension. May be administered with other antihypertensive medications.

Cautions and Warnings

Do not take trichlormethiazide if you are allergic or sensitive to it, to other diuretics, or to sulfa drugs. Some diuretics contain tartrazine, a substance that can cause allergic reactions, especially if you are allergic to aspirin.

Although diuretics have been used to treat specific conditions in pregnancy, unsupervised use by pregnant women should be avoided. Trichlormethiazide can cross the placental barrier and pass into the unborn child, creating the potential for problems. Diuretics are also found in the breast milk of nursing mothers.

Use trichlormethiazide with caution if you suffer from kidney or liver disease.

Trichlormethiazide may activate or worsen gout or lupus (systemic lupus erythematosus).

Trichlormethiazide will increase urination, so you should take it early in the day.

To avoid upset stomach, take the pills with food or milk.

Possible Side Effects

Trichlormethiazide may cause an electrolyte imbalance (potassium loss) in the body. *Signs of low potassium levels* are: dryness of the mouth; thirst; weakness; lethargy; drowsiness; restlessness; muscle pains or cramps; gout; muscle fatigue; decreased frequency of urination and amount of urine; abnormal heart rate; stomach upset (including nausea and vomiting).

To treat this, potassium supplements are available in the form of tablets, liquids, or powders; or your doctor may suggest increased consumption of potassium-rich foods such as bananas, citrus fruits, melons, and tomatoes.

Possible Adverse Effects

Loss of appetite; stomach upset; nausea; vomiting; cramping; diarrhea; constipation; dizziness; headache; tingling of the toes and fingers; restlessness; changes in blood composition; sensitivity to sunlight; rash; itching; fever; difficulty in breathing; allergic reactions; dizziness when rising quickly from a sitting or lying position; muscle spasms; weakness; blurred vision. Rare incidents of impotence have also been reported.

Drug Interactions

Trichlormethiazide may make the action of other blood-pressure-lowering drugs more effective. This is almost always a beneficial action, but your doctor may want to lower your dosage of the other antihypertensive drug.

The possibility of developing imbalances in body fluids and electrolytes is increased if you take certain medications—such as digitalis or adrenal corticosteroids—while you take trichlormethiazide.

If you are taking an oral antidiabetic drug and begin taking trichlormethiazide, the antidiabetic dose may have to be adjusted. Insulin requirements may also be affected.

Lithium carbonate should not be taken with diuretics because the combination may increase the risk of lithium toxicity.

If you are taking trichlormethiazide, avoid over-the-counter medications for the treatment of coughs, colds, and allergies, which may contain stimulants that raise your blood pressure. If you are unsure about which contain stimulants, ask your doctor or pharmacist.

Usual Dose

2 to 4 mg. daily.

Overdosage

Symptoms are increased fatigue, confusion, dizziness, nausea, lethargy, and coma. If you think you are experiencing an overdose, contact your doctor immediately, or go to a hospital emergency room. ALWAYS bring the medicine bottle with you.

Generic Name
Whole Root Rauwolfia

Brand Names

Hiwolfia
Raudixin
Rauserpin
Rauval
Rauverid
Rawfola
Ru-Hy-T
Serfolia
Wolfina
(Also available in generic form)

Type of Drug

Antiadrenergic agent

Prescribed for

The treatment of hypertension—either alone or with other antihypertensive medications.

Cautions and Warnings

Do not stop taking whole root rauwolfia unless directed to do so by your doctor.

Use with extreme caution if you suffer from depression, since whole root rauwolfia may induce severe depression that may persist for several months after you stop taking it. Notify your doctor if you experience any changes in mood or sleep habits, or continual severe stomach pain.

Avoid cough, cold, or allergy medications except when they are approved by your doctor or pharmacist.

If dizziness occurs, avoid suddenly rising from a sitting or reclining position.

Pregnant women should use whole root rauwolfia only when the potential benefits clearly outweigh the unknown potential hazards to the fetus.

Mothers should not breast-feed when taking whole root rauwolfia.

Use whole root rauwolfia with caution if you suffer from kidney or liver disease or have a history of peptic ulcers, ulcerative colitis, or gallstones.

This product may contain tartrazine, a substance found to cause allergic reactions, especially in people allergic to aspirin.

Possible Side Effects

Stuffy nose; dry mouth; dizziness; headache; breathing difficulties; impotence or decreased sex drive; muscle aches; weight gain; breast enlargement; lactation (in females).

Possible Adverse Effects

Nausea; vomiting; loss of appetite; diarrhea; stomach bleeding; chest pain; abnormal heart rhythms; swelling of hands or feet; depression;

fainting; involuntary movements or twitching of the head and neck.

Drug Interactions

Digitalis and quinidine, when used with whole root rauwolfia, may cause abnormal heart rhythms.

MAO inhibitors should be avoided or used with extreme caution.

Whole root rauwolfia, when used with beta blockers, may result in extreme low blood pressure manifested by fainting, vertigo, or dizziness when suddenly rising from a sitting or reclining position.

Usual Dose

Initial dose: 200 to 400 mg. daily in 2 divided doses.

Maintenance dose: 50 to 300 mg. daily in 1 or 2 doses.

Overdosage

Symptoms are changes in consciousness ranging from dizziness to coma; diarrhea; difficulty in breathing; slow heartbeat; flushing of the skin; pupil constriction. If you think you are experiencing an overdose, call your doctor immediately, or go to a hospital emergency room. ALWAYS bring the medicine bottle with you.

SOURCES

Andrews, Gavin, *et al.* "Hypertension: Comparison of Drug and Nondrug Treatments." *British Medical Journal* 284 (22 May 1982): 1523.

Bloxham, C. A., and D. G. Beevers. "Part A, Risk Factors in Essential Hypertension: The Effects of Thiazide Diuretics on Coronary Risk Factors." *Postgraduate Medical Journal* 55 (suppl. 3) (1979): 9–13.

Boyd, J. R., ed. *Facts and Comparisons.* St. Louis: J. B. Lippincott, 1984.

Carney, S., *et al.* "Sodium Restriction and Thiazide Diuretics in the Treatment of Hypertension." *The Medical Journal of Australia* (28 June 1975): 803.

Chobanian, Aram V., and Lorraine Loviglio. *Boston University Medical Center's Heart Risk Book.* New York: Bantam Books, 1982.

Culpepper III, Walter S., *et al.* "Cardiac Status in Juvenile Borderline Hypertension." *Annals of Internal Medicine* 98, no. 1 (January 1983): 1.

Cypress, Beulah K. "Medication Therapy in Office Visits for Hypertension: National Ambulatory Medical Care Survey, 1980." *NCHS Advan-*

cedata, National Center for Health Statistics, U.S. Department of Health and Human Services, no. 80 (22 July 1982).

"The Different Shades of Expert Opinion on Intervention in Approaching HBP Cases." *Medical News*, 15 November 1982.

"Doctors Debate Diet and Drugs for Hypertension." *Modern Medicine*, November 1982: 63.

"Five-Year Findings of the Hypertension Detection and Follow-up Program: Reduction in Mortality of Persons with High Blood Pressure, Including Mild Hypertension." *Journal of the American Medical Association* 242, no. 23 (7 December 1979): 2562.

Foster, Sue B., *et al.* "Influence of Side Effects of Antihypertensive Medication on Patient Behavior." *Cardio-Vascular Nursing* 14, no. 2 (May–June 1978): 9.

Frohlich, Edward D. "Hypertension Drug Rx: When (and What) to Start, Stop, and Add." *Modern Medicine*, December 1982: 52.

Gerber, John G. and Alan S. Nies. "Reactions and Interactions Limiting Use of Antihypertensive Agents." *Journal of Cardiovascular Medicine*, March 1980: 271.

Guyon, Janet. "Rising Concern Over Salt's Effects Stirs Debate, Leads to New Products." *The Wall Street Journal*, 17 December 1982: 29.

A Handbook of Heart Terms. U.S. Department of Health, Education, and Welfare, National Institutes of Health, DHEW Publication no. (NIH) 78–131, undated.

Hart, J. Tudor. "Comparison of Blood Pressure, Sodium Intake, and Other Variables in Offspring With and Without a Family History of High Blood Pressure." *The Lancet*, 4 June 1983: 1245.

"Hypertension and Biofeedback." *Health Facts* (New York: Center for Medical Consumers and Health Care Information, Inc.) 6, no. 31 (December 1981): 3.

Johnson, G. Timothy. "Just Who Is This 'Mr. Fit'?" *New York Daily News*, 22 December 1982: 53.

Johnson, G. Timothy. "Monitor Borderline High Blood Pressure." *New York Daily News*, 27 July 1983: 43.

Johnson, Roger. "Lifestyle Intervention Universal?" *Medical News*, 15 November 1982: 1.

"Juvenile Hypertension." *MD, Medical Newsmagazine* 23, no. 2 (February 1979): 1.

Kaplan, Norman M. "Hypertension: Let Us Not Discard Effective Therapies." Letter to editor, *The New York Times*, 10 October 1982.

Kelleher, Maureen E. "Diuretic Therapy." *The Apothecary*, May/June 1980.

Keyes, Ancel. "Is Overweight a Risk Factor for Coronary Heart Disease?" *Cardiovascular Medicine*, December 1979: 1233.

Laragh, John H. "Hypertension." *Drug Therapy (Hosp)*, January 1980: 47.

Levin, Arthur A. "Treating Mild Hypertension." *Health Facts* (New York: Center for Medical Consumers and Health Care Information, Inc.) 7, no. 35 (April 1982): 2.

Levy, Robert I. "Hypertension Update Reveals Encouraging Trends in Mortality Rates, Public Awareness, and Therapy." *Pharmacy Times*, January 1980: 28.

Lieberman, Ellin. "Children Have Hypertension Too: A Handbook for Pediatric Hypertension." *American Heart Association, Greater Los Angeles Affiliate,* undated.

Liebman, Bonnie. "The Sodium-Hypertension Connection." *Nutrition Action*, December 1982: 5.

Loggie, Jennifer M. H. "Hypertension in the Pediatric Patient: A reappraisal." *The Journal of Pediatrics* 94, no. 5 (May 1979): 685.

McAlister, Neil Harding. "Should We Treat 'Mild' Hypertension?" *Journal of the American Medical Association* 249, no. 3 (21 January 1983): 379.

McCann, Jean. "Surveillance of Millions More at HBP Risk?" *Medical News*, 15 November 1982: 1.

"Mild Hypertension—Are Drugs Appropriate?" *Health Facts* (New York: Center for Medical Consumers and Health Care Information, Inc.) 7, no. 41 (October 1982).

" 'Mild' Hypertension: The Gray Zone Gets More Confusing." *Medical World News*, 20 December 1982: 66.

Mutchie, Kelly D. "Antihypertensive Drugs for Children." *Modern Medicine*, 15 February 1978: 111.

The 1980 Report of the Joint National Committee on Detection, Evaluation, and Treatment of High Blood Pressure. U.S. Department of Health and Human Services, National Institutes of Health, NIH Publication no. 82–1088, December 1981.

The Office Management of Hypertension. KPR Info/Media, New York, for Laboratory Procedures (div. of the Upjohn Company, Michigan), 1976.

O'Brien, Eoin, and Kevin O'Malley. *High Blood Pressure: What It Means For You, and How to Control It.* New York: Arco Publishing, 1982.

Parijs, Jan, *et al.* "Moderate Sodium Restriction and Diuretics in the Treatment of Hypertension." *American Heart Journal* 85, no. 1 (January 1973): 22.

Physicians' Desk Reference. 38th ed. Oradell, New Jersey: Medical Economics Company, 1983.

Report of the Hypertension Task Force, Volume One—General Summary and Recommendations. U.S. Department of Health, Education, and Welfare, National Institutes of Health, NIH Publication no. 79–1623, September 1979.

Rowland, Michael, and Jean Roberts. "Blood Pressure Levels and Hypertension in Persons Ages 6–74 Years: United States, 1976–80." *NCHS Ad vancedata*, National Center for Health Statistics, U.S. Department of Health and Human Services, no. 84 (8 October 1982).

Seligmann, Jean. "Predicting Heart Attacks." *Newsweek*, 22 August 1983: 66.

Shapiro, Alvin P., *et al.* "Behavioral Methods in the Treatment of Hypertension: A Review of Their Clinical Status." *Annals of Internal Medicine* 86, no. 5 (May 1977): 626.

Snider, Arthur J. *A Doctor Discusses: Hypertension (High Blood Pressure).* Chicago: Budlong Press, 1976.

Snider, Arthur J. *A Doctor Discusses: Learning How to Live with Heart Trouble.* Chicago: Budlong Press, 1980.

Solomon, Harold S. "Hypertension." *Office Practice of Medicine,* ed. William T. Branch. Philadelphia: W. B. Saunders, 1982.

Stamler, Rose, and Jeremiah Stamler. " 'Mild' Hypertension: Risks and Strategy for Control." *Primary Cardiology*, October 1983: 150.

Swales, J. D. "Dietary Salt and Hypertension." *The Lancet* 31 (May 1980): 1177.

"TM Has Limitations in Hypertension Therapy." *Modern Medicine* 30 (May 1977).

Taking Your Own Blood Pressure. Ritter-Tycos (div. of Sybron Corp., N.C.) 1983.

Traub, Yehuda M. "New Antihypertensive Agents." *Hospital Formulary,* May 1980: 175.

"Treatment Reduces Deaths from Hypertension." *Science* 206 (21 December 1979): 1386.

Special appreciation to Robert Friedman.

INDEX OF GENERIC AND BRAND NAME DRUGS

Generic drugs are printed in **boldface** type.

ABOUT THE MEDICAL CONSULTANT

HAROLD S. SOLOMON M.D. is Assistant Professor of Medicine at the Harvard Medical School, where he has been a faculty member since 1969. Currently, Dr. Solomon is director of HealthStyle, a heart attack prevention program developed at Beth Israel and Brigham and Women's Hospital in 1979. He is former Director of the Hypertension Clinic at Peter Bent Brigham Hospital and the author of over forty scientific and medical reports on high blood pressure, heart disease, obesity, and health risk reduction.

Dr. Solomon attended the Medical College of Georgia at the University of Georgia and trained in internal medicine at Vanderbilt University and the Harvard Medical School. He lives with his wife and two children in Boston.

SPECIAL
MONEY SAVING
OFFER

---

*Now you can have an up-to-date listing of
Bantam's hundreds of titles plus take advantage
of our unique and exciting bonus book offer. A
special offer which gives you the opportunity to
purchase a Bantam book for only 50¢. Here's
how!*

*By ordering any five books at the regular price
per order, you can also choose any other single
book listed (up to a $4.95 value) for just 50¢.
Some restrictions do apply, but for further details why not send for Bantam's listing of titles
today!*

*Just send us your name and address plus 50¢
to defray the postage and handling costs.*

BANTAM BOOKS, INC.
Dept. FC, 414 East Golf Road, Des Plaines, Ill 60016

Mr./Mrs./Miss/Ms. _____
(please print)

Address _____

City_____ State_____ Zip_____

FC—3/84

How's Your Health?

Bantam publishes a line of informative books, written by top experts to help you toward a healthier and happier life.

We Deliver!
And So Do These Bestsellers.